The Definitive Guide to Dash Seafood Recipes

Enjoy Every Fish Meal with a Collection of Super Easy Recipes for Busy People

I0135229

Naomi Hudson

Table of contents

Lemon Pepper and Salmon

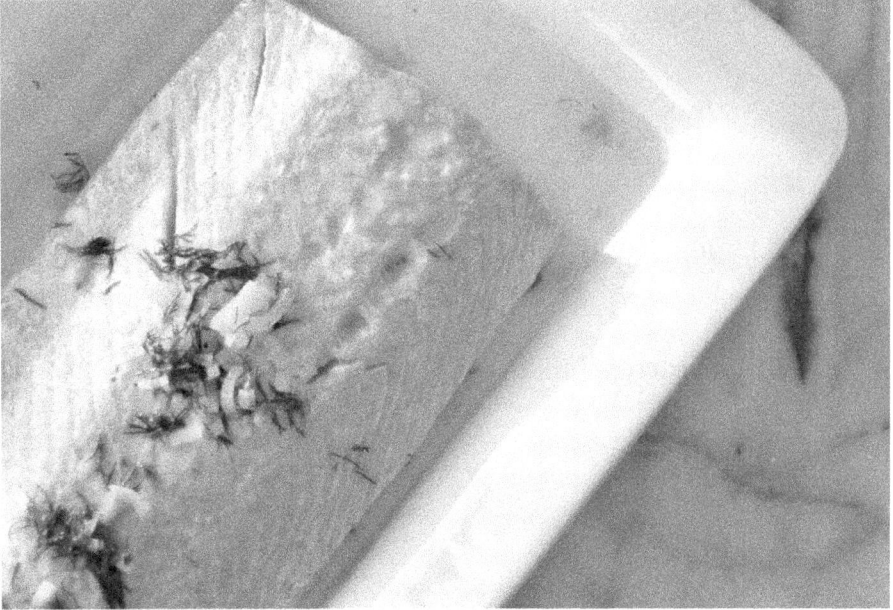

Serving: 3

Prep Time: 5 minute

Cook Time: 6 minutes

Ingredients:

- ¾ cup water

- Few sprigs of parsley, basil, tarragon, basil 1 pound of salmon, skin on teaspoons ghee

- ¼ teaspoon salt

- ½ teaspoon pepper

- ½ lemon, thinly sliced

- 1 whole carrot, julienned

How To:

1. Set your pot to Sauté mode and water and herbs.
2. Place a steamer rack inside your pot and place salmon.
3. Drizzle the ghee on top of the salmon and season with salt and pepper.
4. Cover lemon slices.
5. Lock the lid and cook on high for 3 minutes.
6. Release the pressure naturally over 10 minutes.
7. Transfer the salmon to a serving platter.
8. Set your pot to Sauté mode and add vegetables.
9. Cook for 1-2 minutes.
10. Serve with vegetables and salmon.
11. Enjoy!

Nutrition (Per Serving)

Calories: 464

Fat: 34g

Carbohydrates: 3g

Protein: 34g

Simple Sautéed Garlic and Parsley Scallops

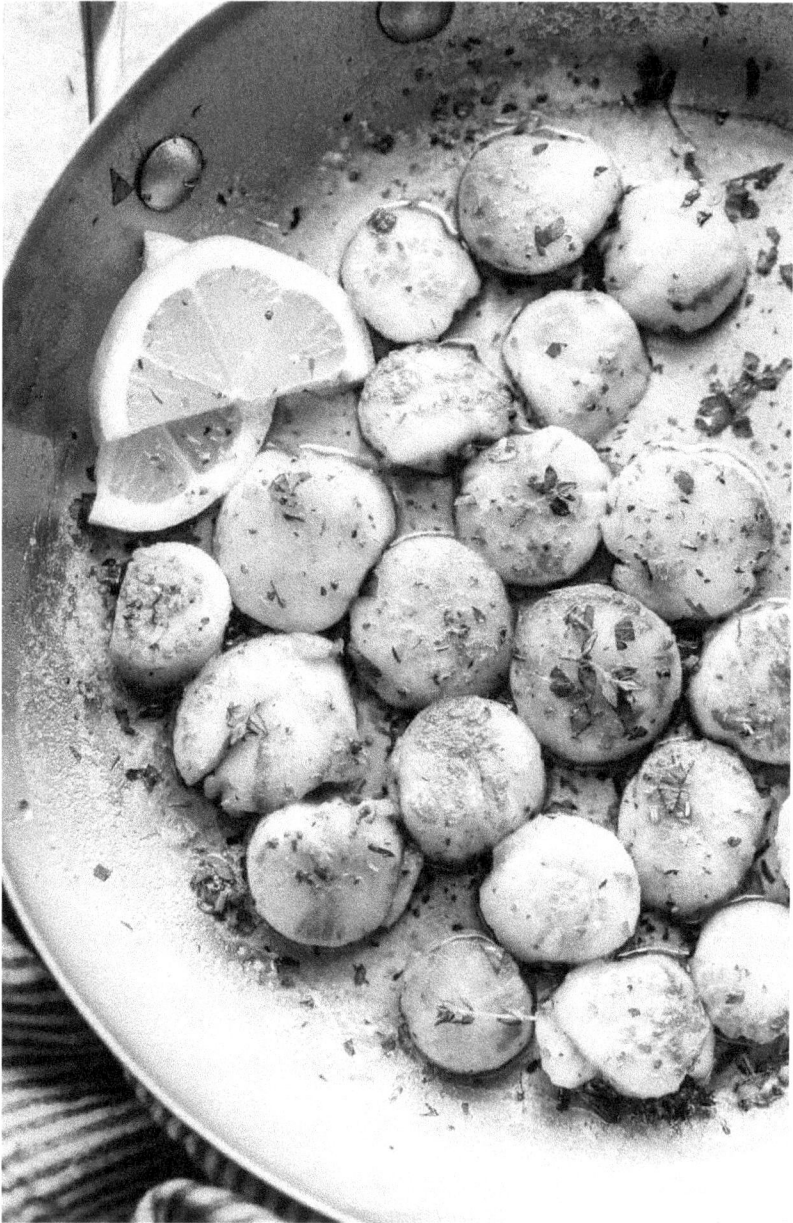

Serving: 4

Prep Time: 5 minutes

Cook Time: 25 minutes

Ingredients:

- 8 tablespoons almond butter

- 2 garlic cloves, minced

- 16 large sea scallops

- Sunflower seeds and pepper to taste

- 1 ½ tablespoons olive oil

How To:

1.   Seasons scallops with sunflower seeds and pepper.

2.   Take a skillet, place it over medium heat, add oil and let it heat up.

3.   Sauté scallops for two minutes per side, repeat until all scallops are cooked.

4.   Add almond butter to the skillet and let it melt.

5.   Stir in garlic and cook for quarter-hour .

6.   Return scallops to skillet and stir to coat.

7.   Serve and enjoy!

Nutrition (Per Serving)

Calories: 417

Fat: 31g

Net Carbohydrates: 5g

Protein: 29g

Salmon and Cucumber Platter

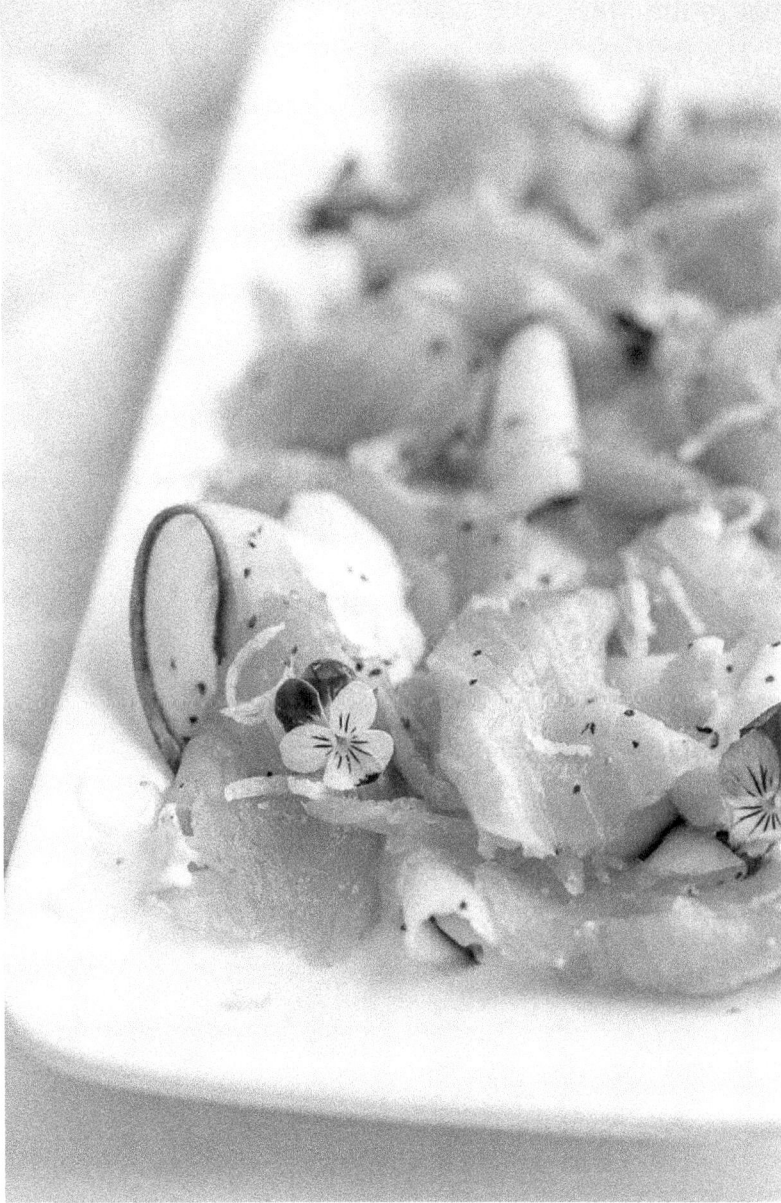

Serving: 4

Prep Time: 10 minutes

Cook Time: nil

Ingredients:

- 2 cucumbers, cubed

- 2 teaspoons fresh squeezed lemon juice ounces non-fat yogurt teaspoon lemon zest, grated

- Pepper to taste

- teaspoons dill, chopped

- 8 ounces smoked salmon, flaked

How To:

1. Take a bowl and add cucumbers, juice , lemon peel , pepper, dill,salmon, yogurt and toss well.

2. Serve cold.

3.   Enjoy!

Nutrition (Per Serving)

Calories: 242

Fat: 3g

Carbohydrates: 3g

Protein: 3g

Tuna Paté

Serving: 4

Prep Time: 10 minutes

Cook Time: nil

Ingredients:

- ounces canned tuna, drained and flaked teaspoons fresh lemon juice 1 teaspoon onion, minced

- ounces low-fat cream cheese

- ¼ cup parsley, chopped

How To:

1.   Take a bowl and blend in tuna, cheese , juice , parsley, onion and stir well.

2.   Serve cold and enjoy!

Nutrition (Per Serving)

Calories: 172

Fat: 2g

Carbohydrates: 8g

Protein: 4g

Cinnamon Salmon

Serving: 4

Prep Time: 10 minutes

Cook Time: 10 minutes

Ingredients:

- 2 salmon fillets, boneless and skin on

- Pepper to taste

- 1 tablespoon cinnamon powder

- 1 tablespoon organic olive oil

How To:

1.   Take a pan and place it over medium heat, add oil and let it heat up.

2.   Add pepper, cinnamon and stir.

3.   Add salmon, skin side up and cook for five minutes on each side .

4.   Divide between plates and serve.

5.   Enjoy!

Nutrition (Per Serving)

Calories: 220

Fat: 8g

Carbohydrates: 11g

Protein: 8g

Scallop and Strawberry Mix

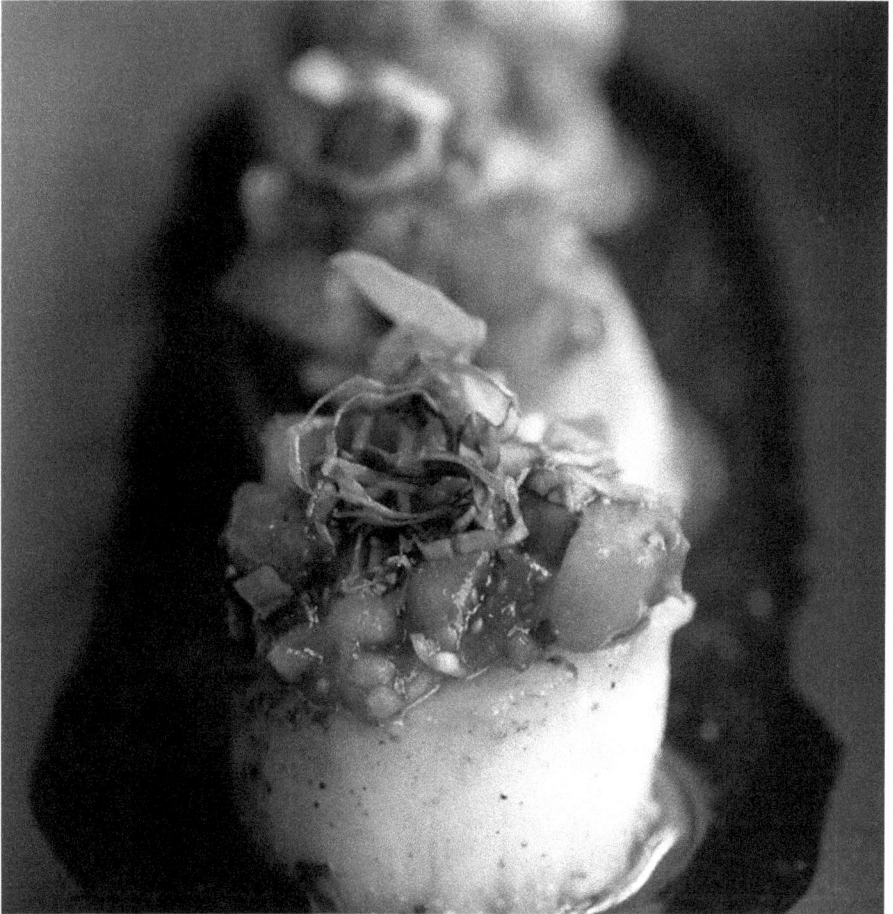

Serving: 4

Prep Time: 10 minutes

Cook Time: 6 minutes

Ingredients:

- ounces scallops

- ½ cup Pico De Gallo

- ½ cup strawberries, chopped

- 1 tablespoon lime juice

Pepper to taste

How To:

1.	Take a pan and place it over medium heat, add scallops and cook for 3 minutes on each side .

2.	Remove heat.

3.	Take a bowl and add strawberries, juice , Pico De Gallo, scallops, pepper and toss well.

4.	Serve and enjoy!

Nutrition (Per Serving)

Calories: 169

Fat: 2g

Carbohydrates: 8g

Protein: 13g

Salmon and Orange Dish

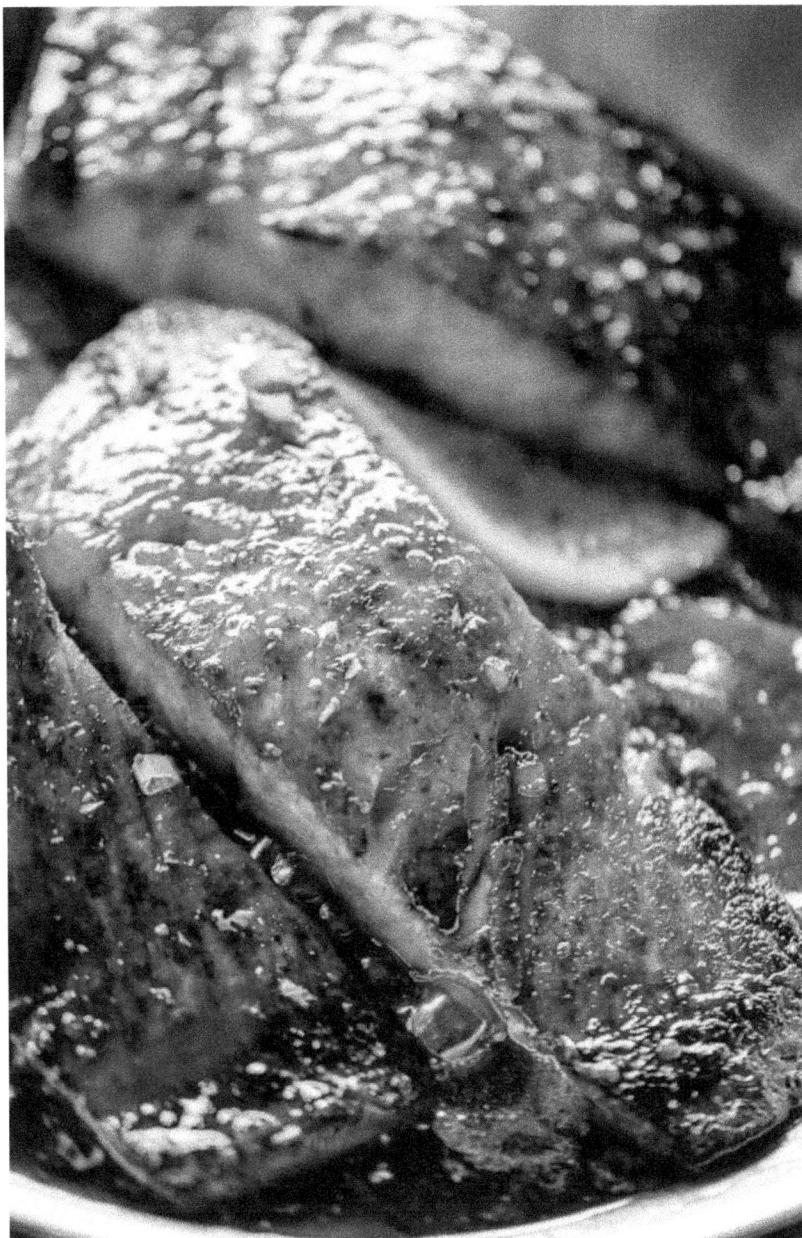

Serving: 4

Prep Time: 10 minute

Cook Time: 15 minutes

Ingredients:

- salmon fillets

- cup orange juice

- tablespoons arrowroot and water mixture 1 teaspoon orange peel, grated 1 teaspoon black pepper

How To:

1. Add the listed ingredients to your pot.
2. Lock the lid and cook on high for 12 minutes.
3. Release the pressure naturally.
4. Serve and enjoy!

Nutrition (Per Serving)

Calories:583

Fat: 20g

Carbohydrates: 71g

Protein: 33g

Mesmerizing Coconut Haddock

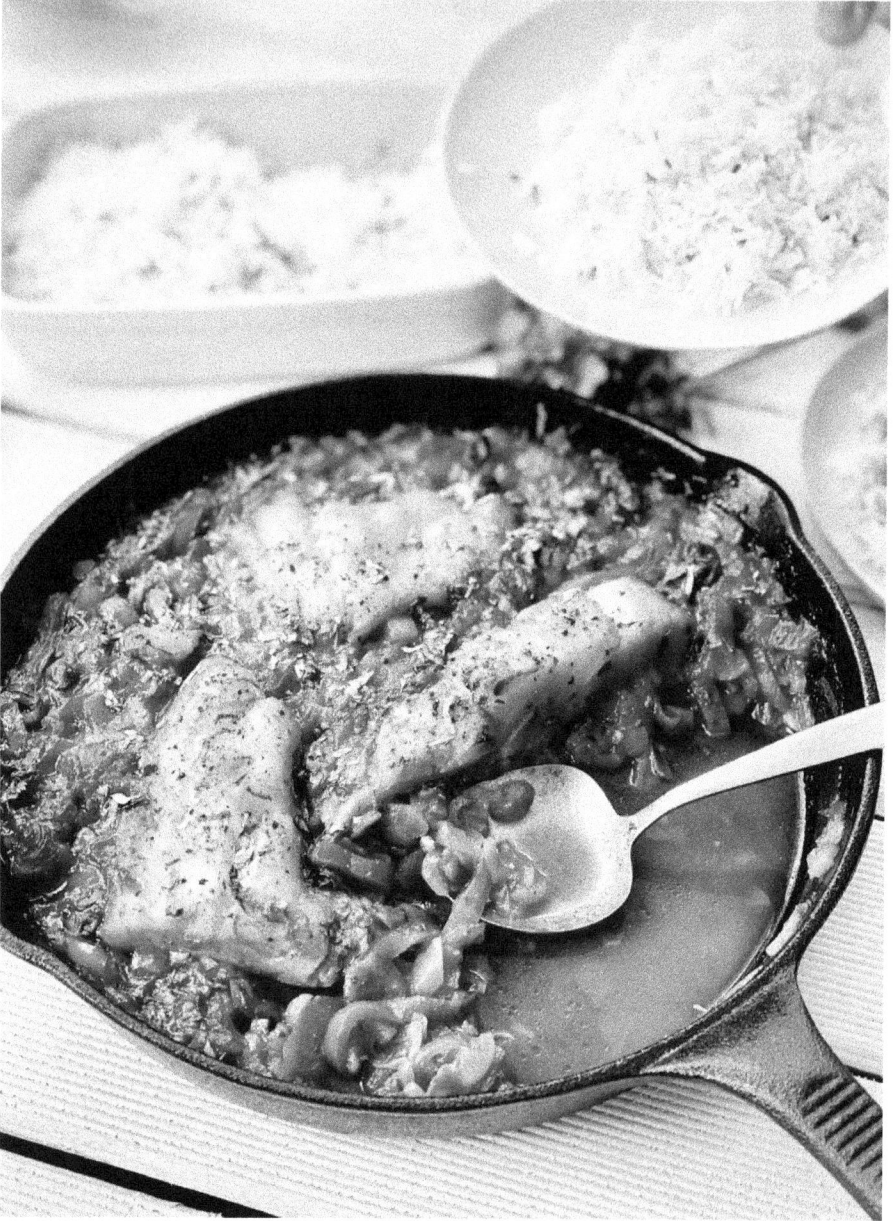

Serving: 3

Prep Time: 10 minutes

Cook Time: 12 minutes

Ingredients:

- Haddock fillets, 5 ounces each, boneless 2 tablespoons coconut oil, melted

- 1 cup coconut, shredded and unsweetened

- ¼ cup hazelnuts, ground Sunflower seeds to taste

How To:

1. Pre-heat your oven to 400 degrees F.
2. Line a baking sheet with parchment paper.
3. Keep it on the side.
4. Pat fish fillets with towel and season with sunflower seeds.
5. Take a bowl and stir in hazelnuts and shredded coconut.
6. Drag fish fillets through the coconut mix until each side are coated well.
7. Transfer to baking dish.
8. Brush with copra oil .

9.   Bake for about 12 minutes until flaky.

10.   Serve and enjoy!

Nutrition (Per Serving)

Calories: 299

Fat: 24g

Carbohydrates: 1g

Protein: 20g

Asparagus and Lemon Salmon Dish

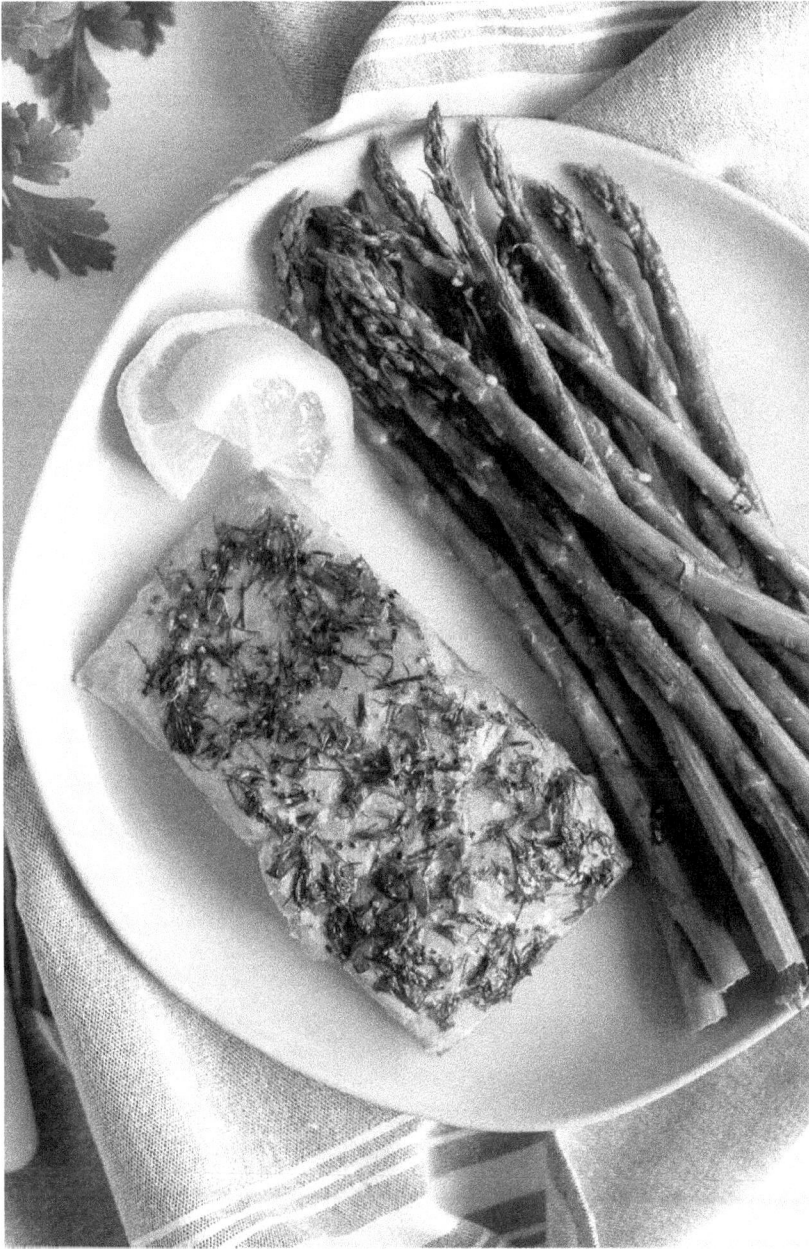

Serving: 3

Prep Time: 5 minutes

Cook Time: 15 minutes

Ingredients:

- 2 salmon fillets, 6 ounces each, skin on Sunflower seeds to taste

- 1-pound asparagus, trimmed 2 cloves garlic, minced tablespoons almond butter ¼ cup cashew cheese

How To:

Pre-heat your oven to 400 degrees F.

Line a baking sheet with oil.

Take a kitchen towel and pat your salmon dry, season as needed.

1.   Put salmon onto the baking sheet and arrange asparagus around it.

2.   Place a pan over medium heat and melt almond butter.

3.   Add garlic and cook for 3 minutes until garlic browns slightly.

4.   Drizzle sauce over salmon.

5.   Sprinkle salmon with cheese and bake for 12 minutes until salmon looks cooked all the way and is flaky.

6.   Serve and enjoy!

Nutrition (Per Serving)

Calories: 434

Fat: 26g

Carbohydrates: 6g

Protein: 42g

Ecstatic "Foiled" Fish

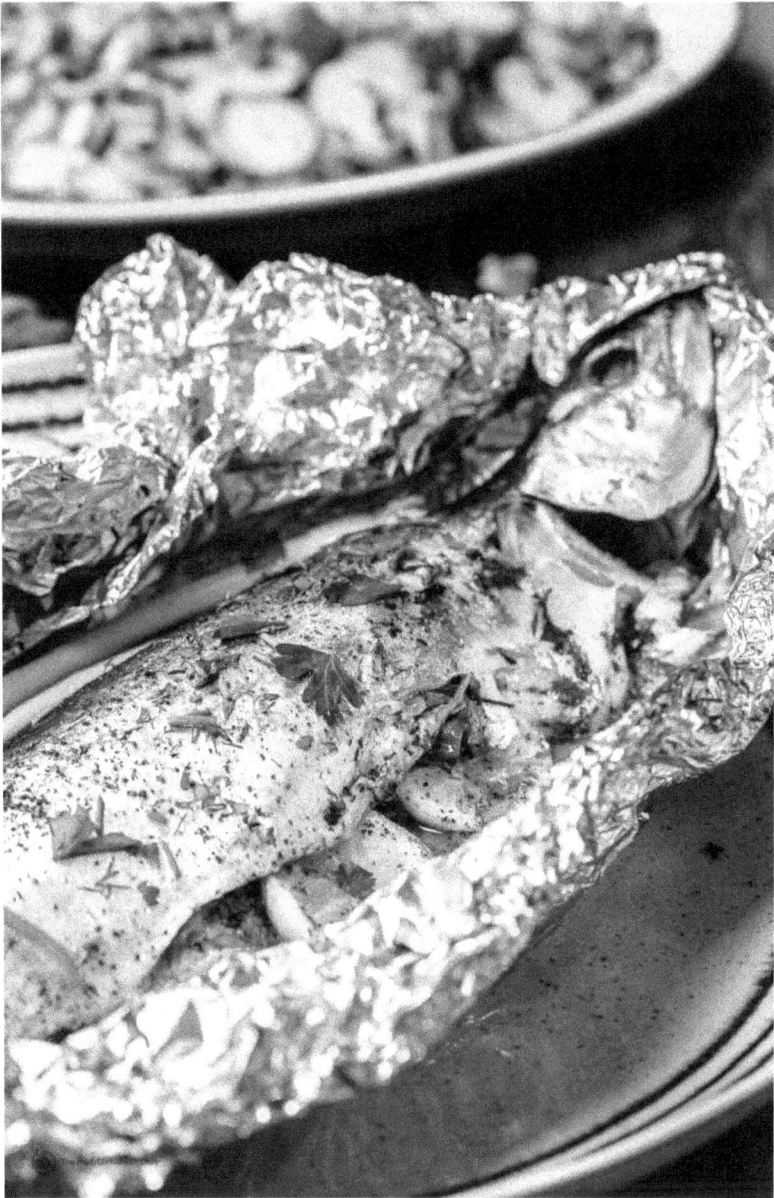

Serving: 4

Prep Time: 20 minutes

Cook Time: 40 minutes

Ingredients:

- 2 rainbow trout fillets

- tablespoon olive oil

- teaspoon garlic salt

- 1 teaspoon ground black pepper

- 1 fresh jalapeno pepper, sliced

- 1 lemon, sliced

How To:

1.   Pre-heat your oven to 400 degrees F.

2. Rinse your fish and pat them dry.

3. Rub the fillets with olive oil, season with some garlic salt and black pepper.

4. Place each of your seasoned fillets on a large sized sheet of aluminum foil.

5. Top it with some jalapeno slices and squeeze the juice from your lemons over your fish.

6. Arrange the lemon slices on top of your fillets.

7. Carefully seal up the edges of your foil and form a nice enclosed packet.

8. Place your packets on your baking sheet.

9. Bake them for about 20 minutes.

10. Once the flakes start to flake off with a fork, the fish is ready!

Nutrition (Per Serving)

Calories: 213

Fat: 10g

Carbohydrates: 8g

Protein: 24g

Brazilian Shrimp Stew

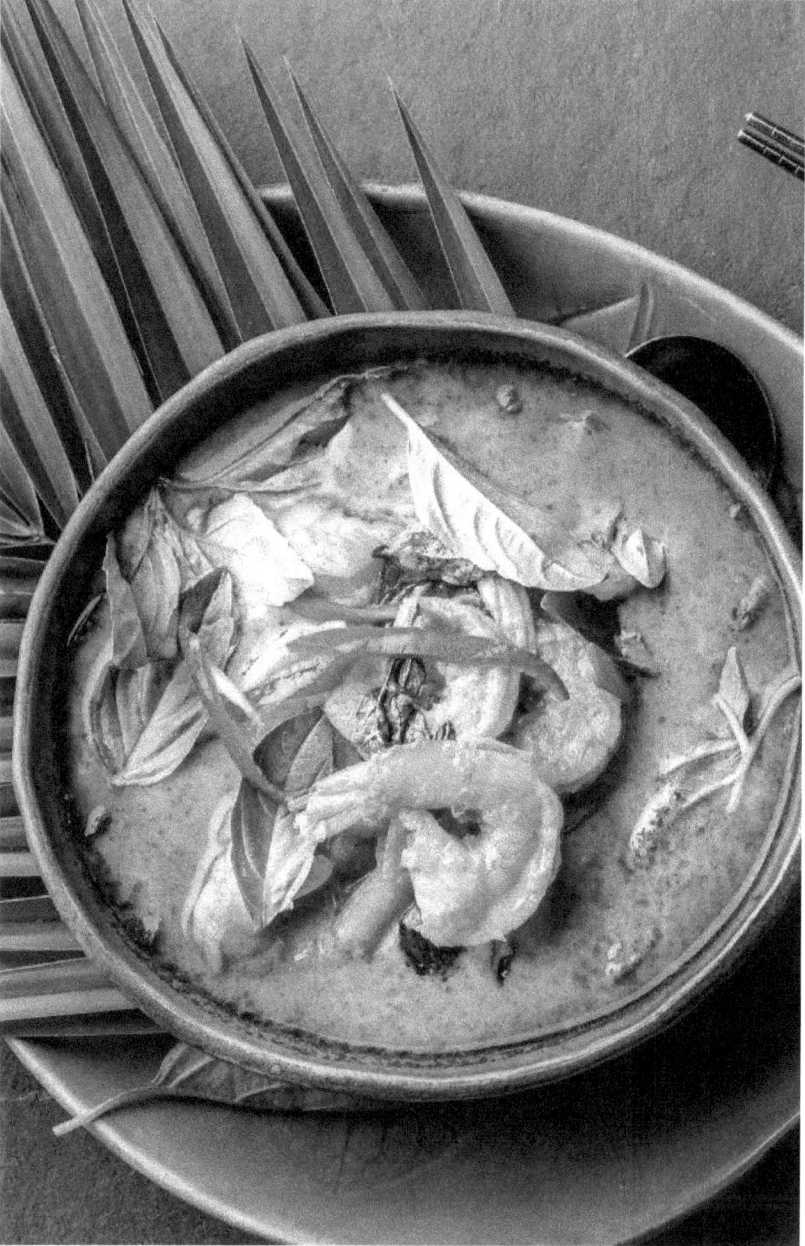

Serving: 4

Prep Time: 20 minutes

Cook Time: 25 minutes

Ingredients:

- Tablespoons lime juice

- 1 ½ tablespoons cumin, ground

- ½ tablespoons paprika

- ½ teaspoons garlic, minced

- ½ teaspoons pepper

- Pounds tilapia fillets, cut into bits

- 1 large onion, chopped

- Large bell peppers, cut into strips

- 1 can (14 ounces) tomato, drained

- 1 can (14 ounces) coconut milk handful of cilantros, chopped

How To:

1.   Take a large sized bowl and add lime juice, cumin, paprika, garlic, pepper and mix well.

2.   Add tilapia and coat it up.

3.   Cover and allow to marinate for 20 minutes.

4.   Set your Instant Pot to Sauté mode and add olive oil.

5.   Add onions and cook for 3 minutes until tender.

6.   Add pepper strips, tilapia, and tomatoes to a skillet.

7.   Pour coconut milk and cover, simmer for 20 minutes.

8.   Add cilantro during the final few minutes.

9.   Serve and enjoy!

Nutrition (Per Serving)

Calories: 471

Fat: 44g

Carbohydrates: 13g

Protein: 12g

Inspiring Cajun Snow Crab

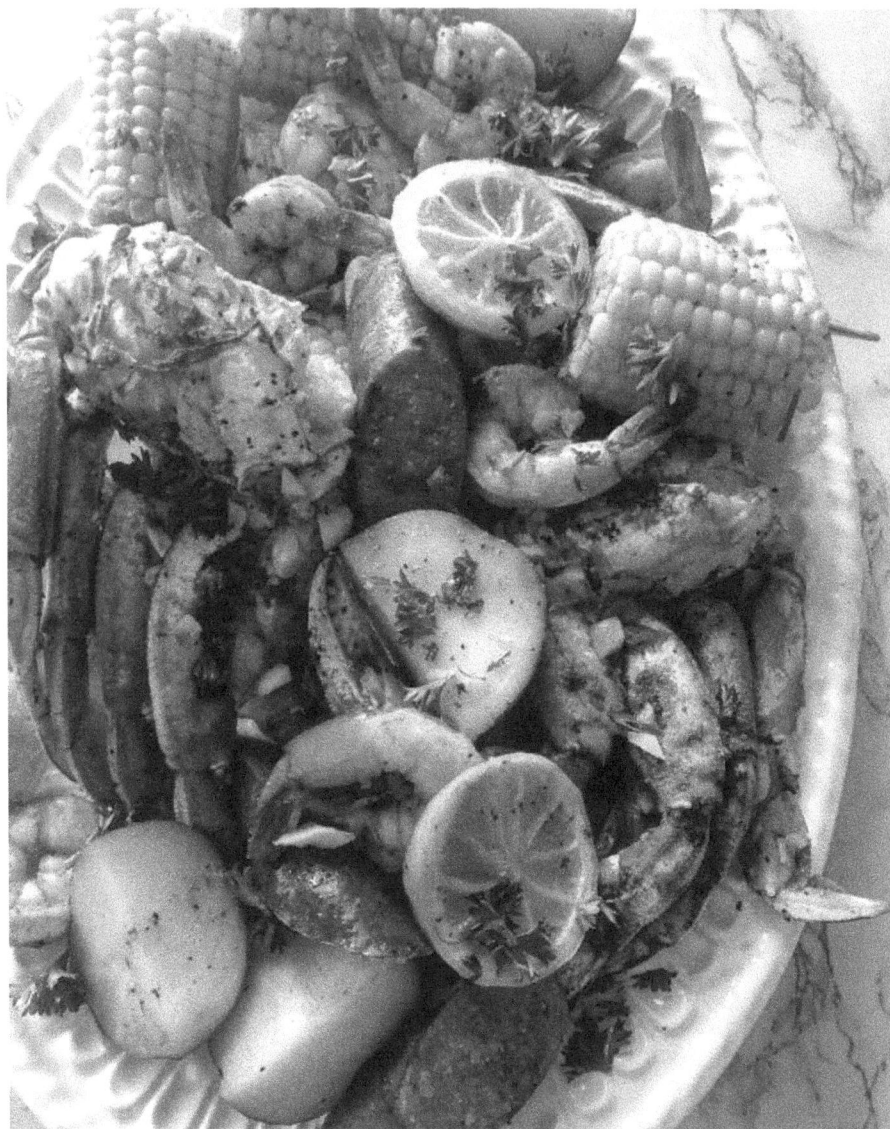

Serving: 2

Prep Time: 10 minutes

Cook Time: 10 minutes

Ingredients:

- 1 lemon, fresh and quartered tablespoons

- Cajun seasoning

- Bay leaves

- Snow crab legs, precooked and defrosted Golden ghee

How To:

1.   Take a large pot and fill it about halfway with sunflower seeds and water.

2.   Bring the water to a boil.

3.   Squeeze lemon juice into the pot and toss in remaining lemon quarters.

4.   Add bay leaves and Cajun seasoning.

5.   Season for 1 minute.

6.   Add crab legs and boil for 8 minutes (make sure to keep them submerged the whole time).

7.   Melt ghee in microwave and use as dipping sauce, enjoy!

Nutrition (Per Serving)

Calories: 643

Fat: 51g

Carbohydrates: 3g

Protein: 41g

Grilled Lime Shrimp

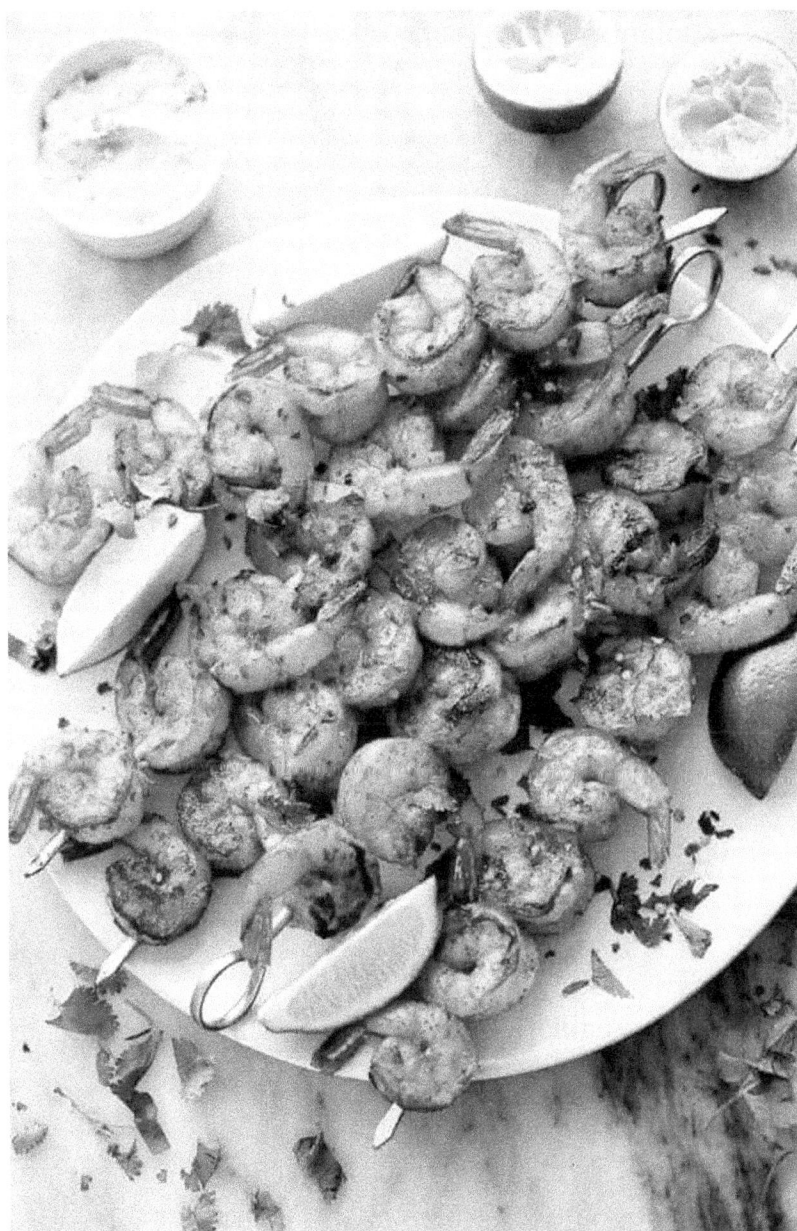

Serving: 8

Prep Time: 25 minutes

Cook Time: 5 minutes

Ingredients:

- 1-pound medium shrimp, peeled and deveined

- 1 lime, juiced

- ½ cup olive oil

- Cajun seasoning

How To:

1.   Take a re-sealable zip bag and add lime juice, Cajun seasoning, olive oil.

2.   Add shrimp and shake it well, let it marinate for 20 minutes.

3.   Pre-heat your outdoor grill to medium heat.

4.   Lightly grease the grate.

5.   Remove shrimp from marinade and cook for 2 minutes per side.

6.   Serve and enjoy!

Nutrition (Per Serving)

Calories: 188

Fat: 3g

Net Carbohydrates: 1.2g

Protein: 13g

Calamari Citrus

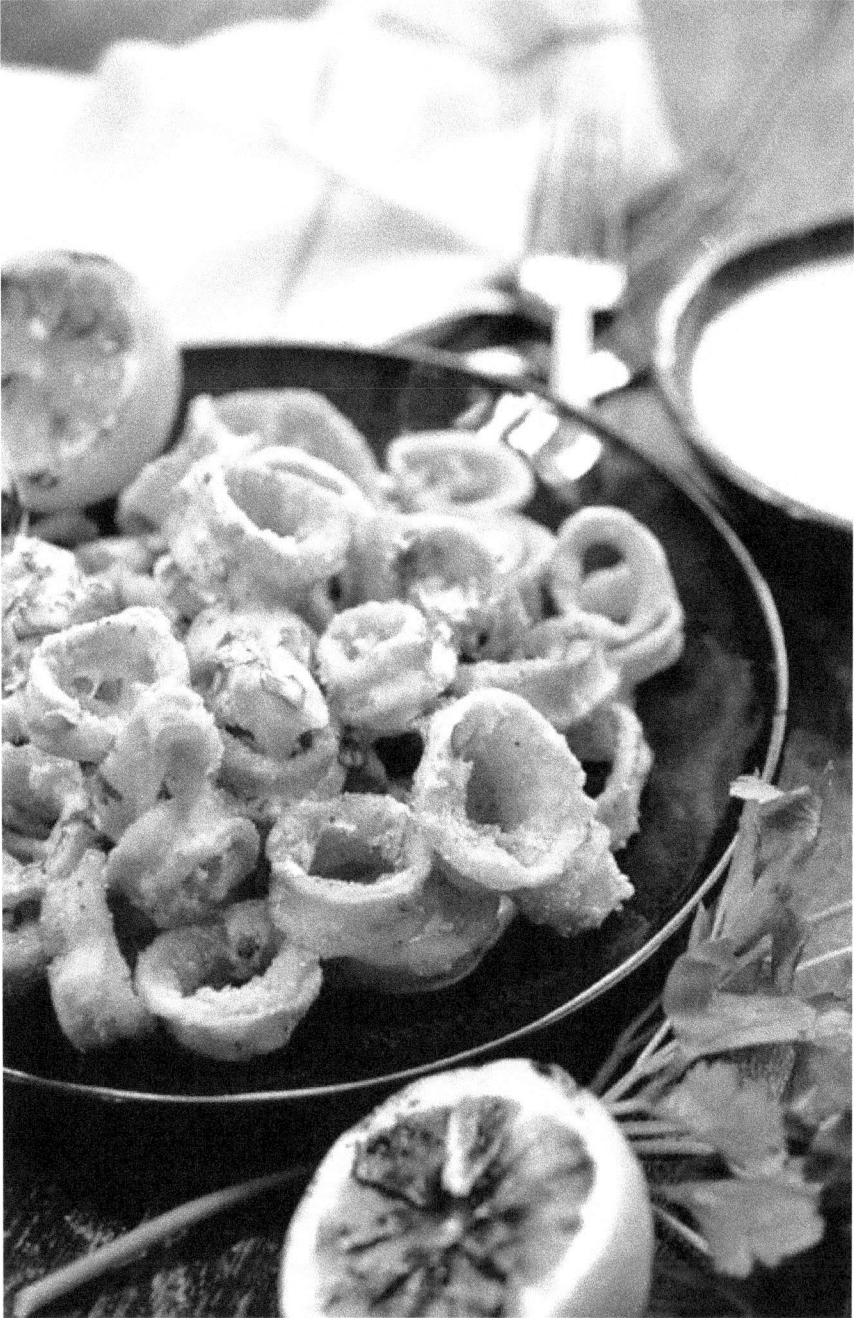

Serving: 4

Prep Time: 10 minutes

Cook Time: 5 minutes

Ingredients:

- 1 lime, sliced

- lemon, sliced

- Pounds calamari tubes and tentacles, sliced

- Pepper to taste

- ¼ cup olive oil

- garlic cloves, minced

- tablespoons lemon juice

- orange, peeled and cut into segments

- tablespoons cilantro, chopped

How To:

1.   Take a bowl and add calamari, pepper, lime slices, lemon slices, orange slices, garlic, oil, cilantro, lemon juice and toss well.

2.   Take a pan and place it over medium-high heat.

3.   Add calamari mix and cook for 5 minutes.

4.   Divide into bowls and serve.

5.   Enjoy!

Nutrition (Per Serving)

Calories: 190

Fat: 2g

Net Carbohydrates: 11g

Protein: 14g

Spiced Up Salmon

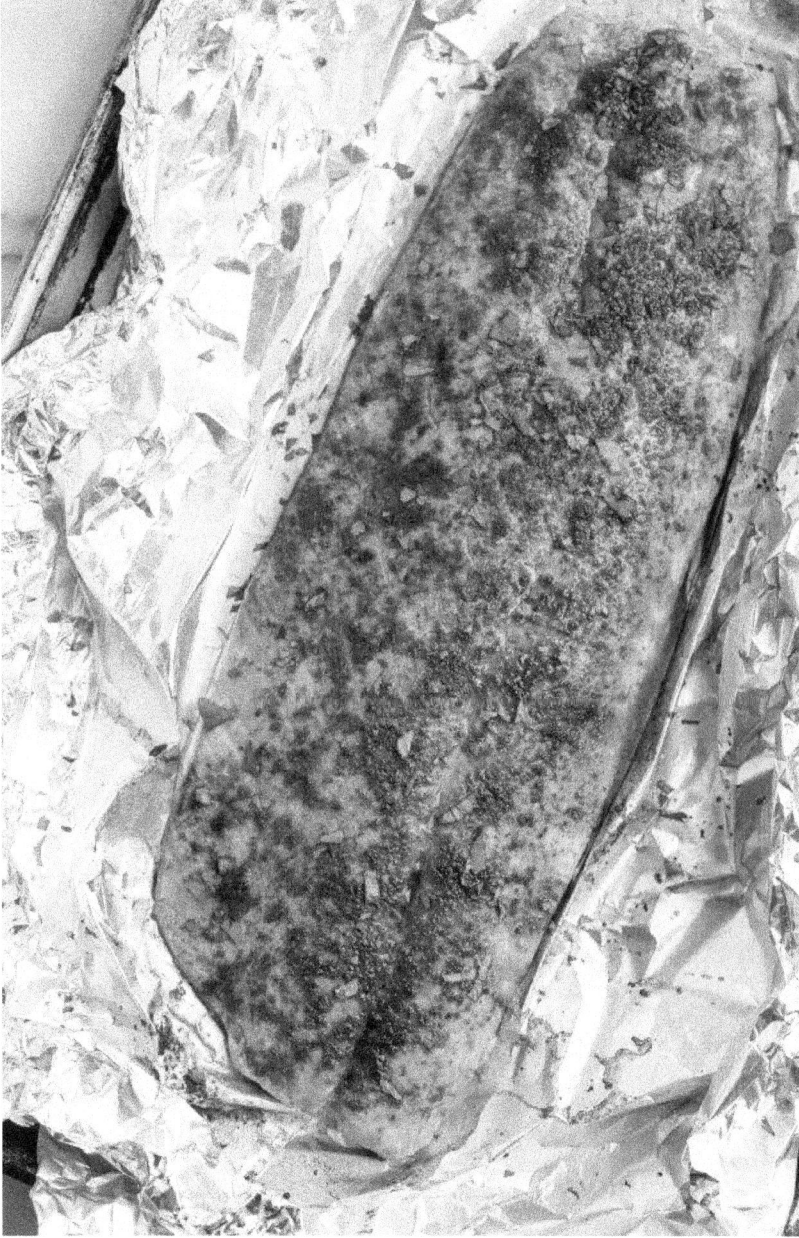

Serving: 4

Prep Time: 10 minutes

Cook Time: 10 minutes

Ingredients:

- Salmon fillets

- 2 tablespoons olive oil

- 1 teaspoon cumin, ground

- 1 teaspoon sweet paprika

- 1 teaspoon chili powder

- ½ teaspoon garlic powder

- Pinch of pepper

How To:

1. Take a bowl and add cumin, paprika, onion, chili powder, garlic powder, pepper and toss well.

2. Rub the salmon in the mixture.

3. Take a pan and place it over medium heat, add oil and let it heat up.

4. Add salmon and cook for 5 minutes, both sides.

5. Divide between plates and serve.

6. Enjoy!

Nutrition (Per Serving)

Calories: 220

Fat: 10g

Net Carbohydrates: 8g

Protein: 10g

Coconut Cream Shrimp

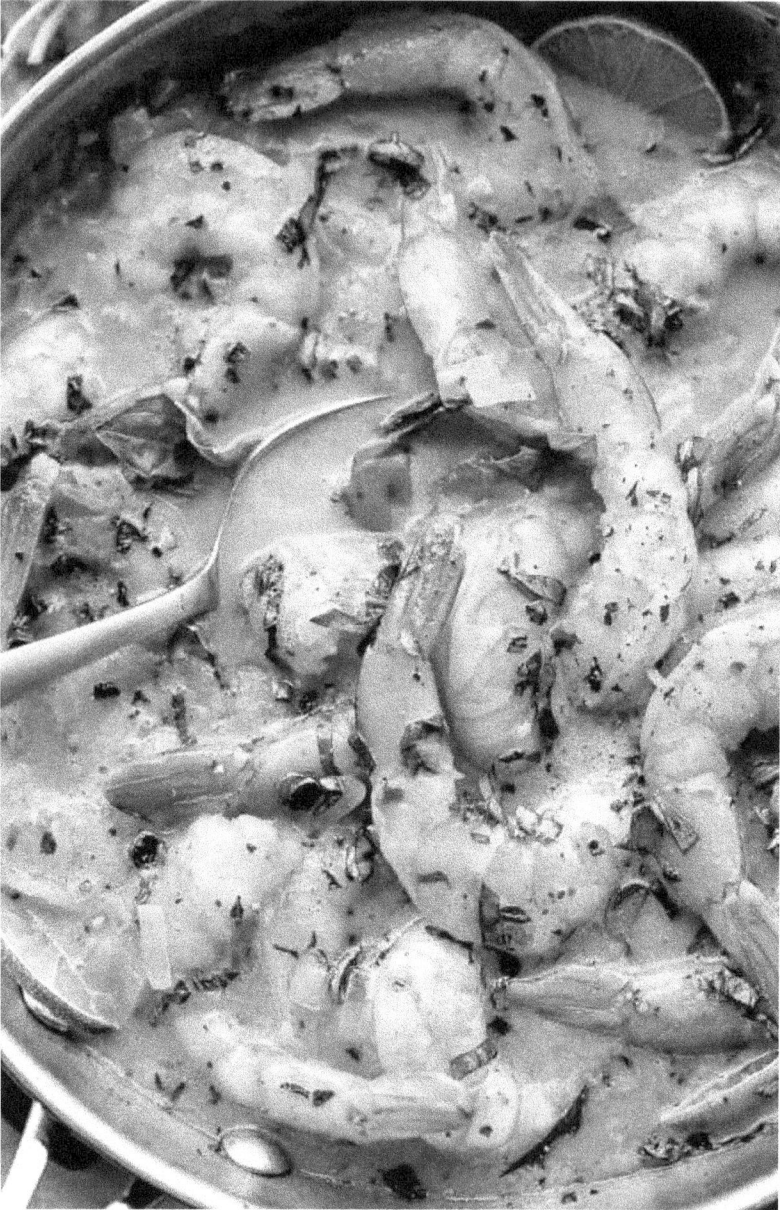

Serving: 4

Prep Time: 10 minutes

Cook Time: nil

Ingredients:

- 1 pound shrimp, cooked , peeled and deveined

- 1 tablespoon coconut cream

- ¼ teaspoon jalapeno, chopped ½ teaspoon lime juice 1 tablespoon parsley, chopped Pinch of pepper

How To:

1.   Take a bowl and add shrimp, cream, jalapeno, lime juice, parsley, pepper.

2.   Toss well and divide into small bowls.

3.   Serve and enjoy!

Nutrition (Per Serving)

Calories: 183

Fat: 5g

Net Carbohydrates: 12g

Protein: 8g

Shrimp and Avocado Platter

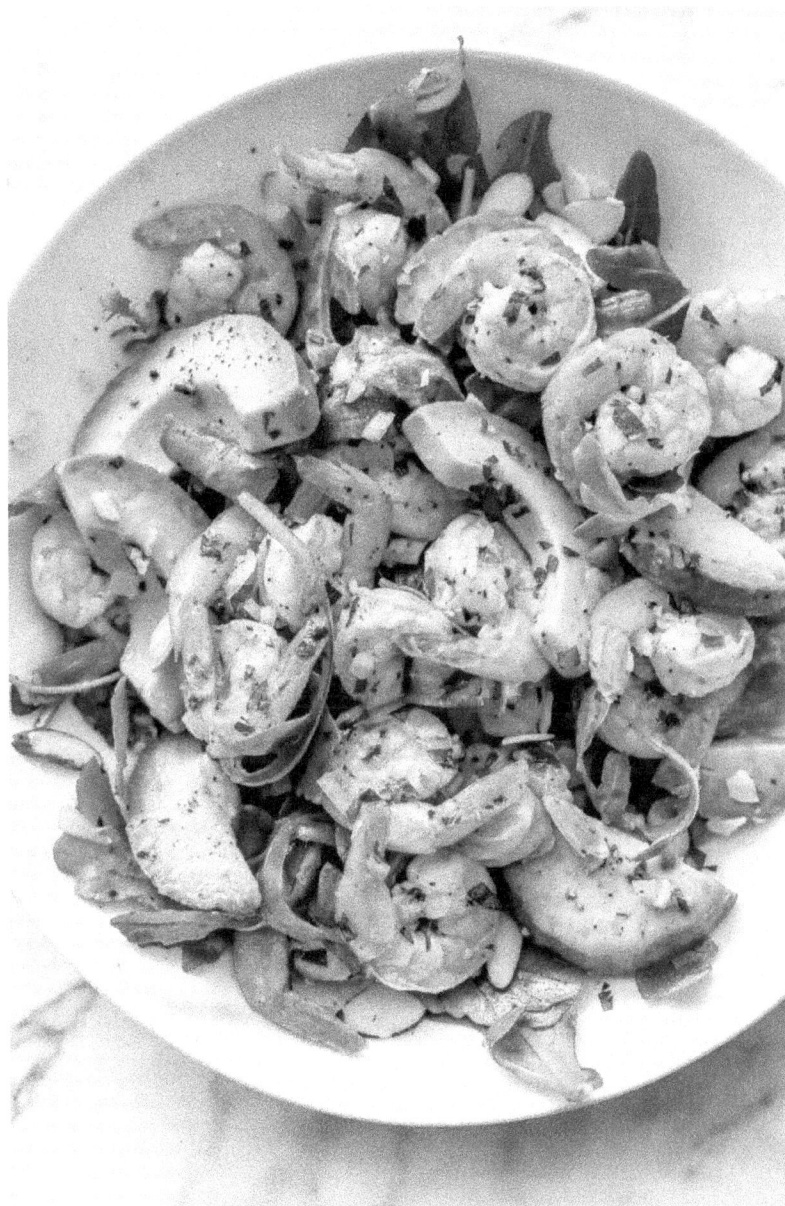

Serving: 8

Prep Time: 10 minutes

Cook Time: nil

Ingredients:

- 2 green onions, chopped

- 2 avocados, pitted, peeled and cut into chunks

- 2 tablespoons cilantro, chopped

- 1 cup shrimp, cooked, peeled and deveined Pinch of pepper

How To:

1.   Take a bowl and add cooked shrimp, avocado, green onions, cilantro, pepper.

2.   Toss well and serve.

3.   Enjoy!

Nutrition (Per Serving)

Calories: 160

Fat: 2g

Net Carbohydrates: 5g

Protein: 6g

Calamari

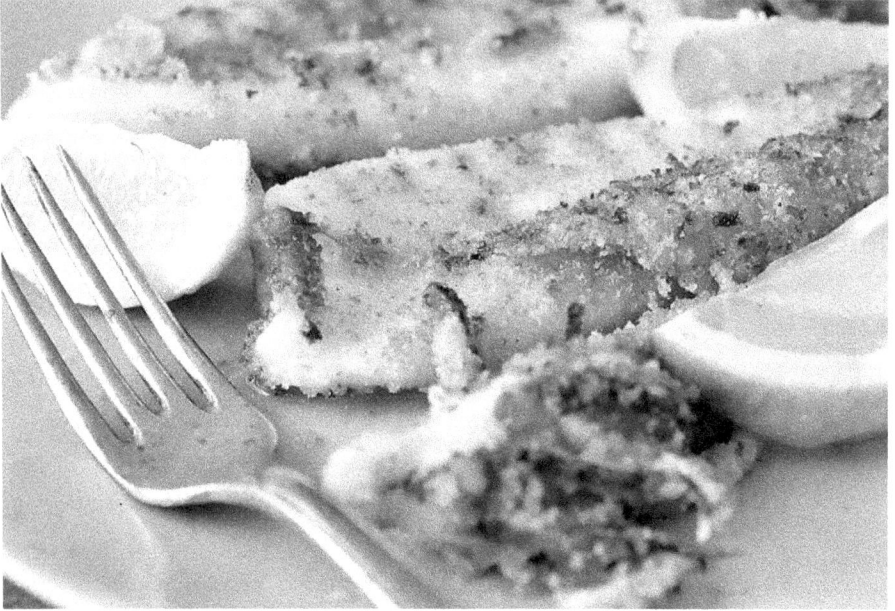

Serving: 4

Prep Time: 10 minutes +1-hour marinating

Cook Time: 8 minutes

Ingredients:

- 2 tablespoons extra virgin olive oil

- 1 teaspoon chili powder

- ½ teaspoon ground cumin

- Zest of 1 lime

- Juice of 1 lime

- Dash of sea sunflower seeds

- ½ pounds squid, cleaned and split open, with tentacles cut into ½ inch rounds

- tablespoons cilantro, chopped

- tablespoons red bell pepper, minced

How To:

1.   Take a medium bowl and stir in olive oil, chili powder, cumin, lime zest, sea sunflower seeds, lime juice and pepper.

2.   Add squid and let it marinade and stir to coat, coat and let it refrigerate for 1 hour

3.   Pre-heat your oven to broil.

4.   Arrange squid on a baking sheet, broil for 8 minutes turn once until tender.

5.   Garnish the broiled calamari with cilantro and red bell pepper.

6.   Serve and enjoy!

Nutrition (Per Serving)

Calories: 159

Fat: 13g

Carbohydrates: 12g

Protein: 3g

Hearty Deep-Fried Prawn and Rice Croquettes

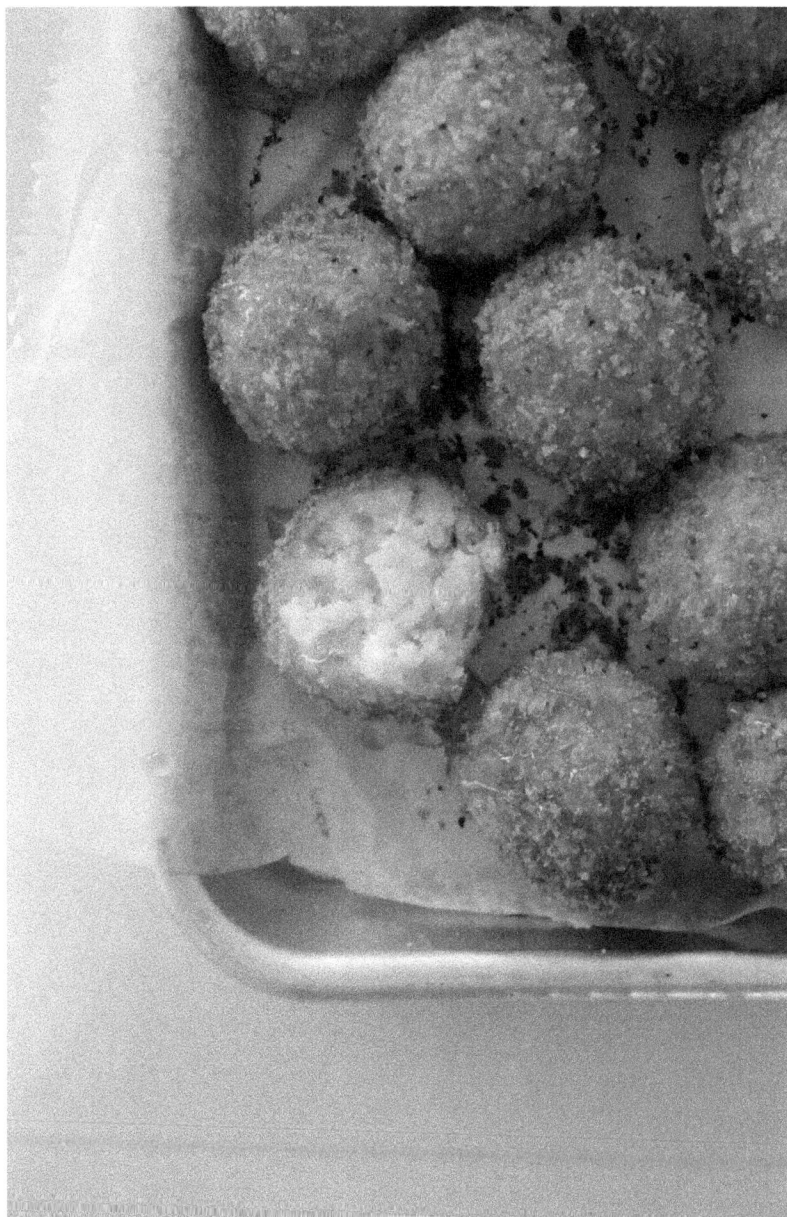

Serving: 8

Prep Time: 25 minute

Cook Time: 13 minutes

Ingredients:

- 2 tablespoons almond butter

- ½ onion, chopped

- ounces shrimp, peeled and chopped

- 2 tablespoons all-purpose flour

- tablespoon white wine

- ½ cup almond milk

- tablespoons almond milk

- cups cooked rice

- 1 tablespoon parmesan, grated

- 1 teaspoon fresh dill, chopped

- 1 teaspoon sunflower seeds

- Ground pepper as needed

- Vegetable oil for frying
- tablespoons all-purpose flour
- 1 whole egg

- ½ cup breadcrumbs

How To:

1.   Take a large skillet and place it over medium heat, add almond butter and let it melt.

2.   Add onion, cook and stir for 5 minutes.

3.   Add shrimp and cook for 1-2 minutes.

4.   Stir in 2 tablespoons flour, white wine, pour in almond milk gradually and cook for 3-5 minutes until the sauce thickens.

5.   Remove white sauce from heat and stir in rice, mix evenly.

6.   Add parmesan, cheese, dill, sunflower seeds, pepper and let it cool for 15 minutes.

7.   Heat oil in large saucepan and bring it to 350 degrees F.

8.   Take a bowl and whisk in egg, spread breadcrumbs on a plate.

9.   Form rice mixture into 8 balls and roll 1 ball in flour, dip in egg and coat with crumbs, repeat with all balls.

10.   Deep fry balls for 3 minutes.

11.   Enjoy!

Nutrition (Per Serving)

Calories: 182

Fat: 7g

Carbohydrates: 21g

Protein: 7g

Easy Garlic Almond butter Shrimp

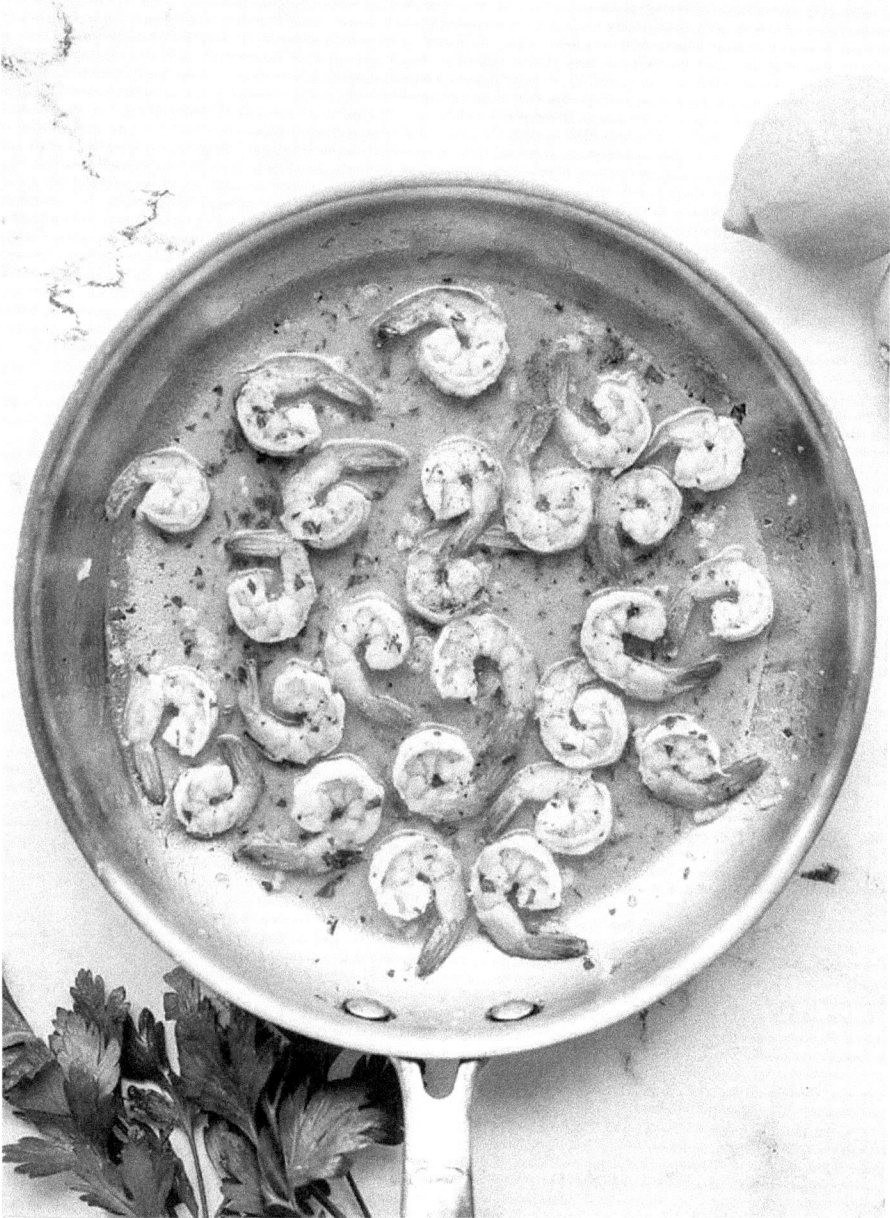

Serving: 4

Prep Time: 15 minutes

Cook Time: 30 minutes

Ingredients:

- pounds shrimp

- 1-2 tablespoons garlic, minced

- ½ cup almond butter

- 1 tablespoon lemon pepper seasoning

- ½ teaspoon garlic powder

How To:

1.   Pre-heat your oven to 300 degrees F.

2.   Take a bowl and mix in garlic and almond butter.

3.   Place shrimp in a pan and dot with almond butter garlic mix.

4. Sprinkle garlic powder and lemon pepper.

5. Bake for 30 minutes.

6. Enjoy!

Nutrition (Per Serving)

Calories: 749

Fat: 30g

Net Carbohydrates: 7g

Protein: 74g

Blackened Tilapia

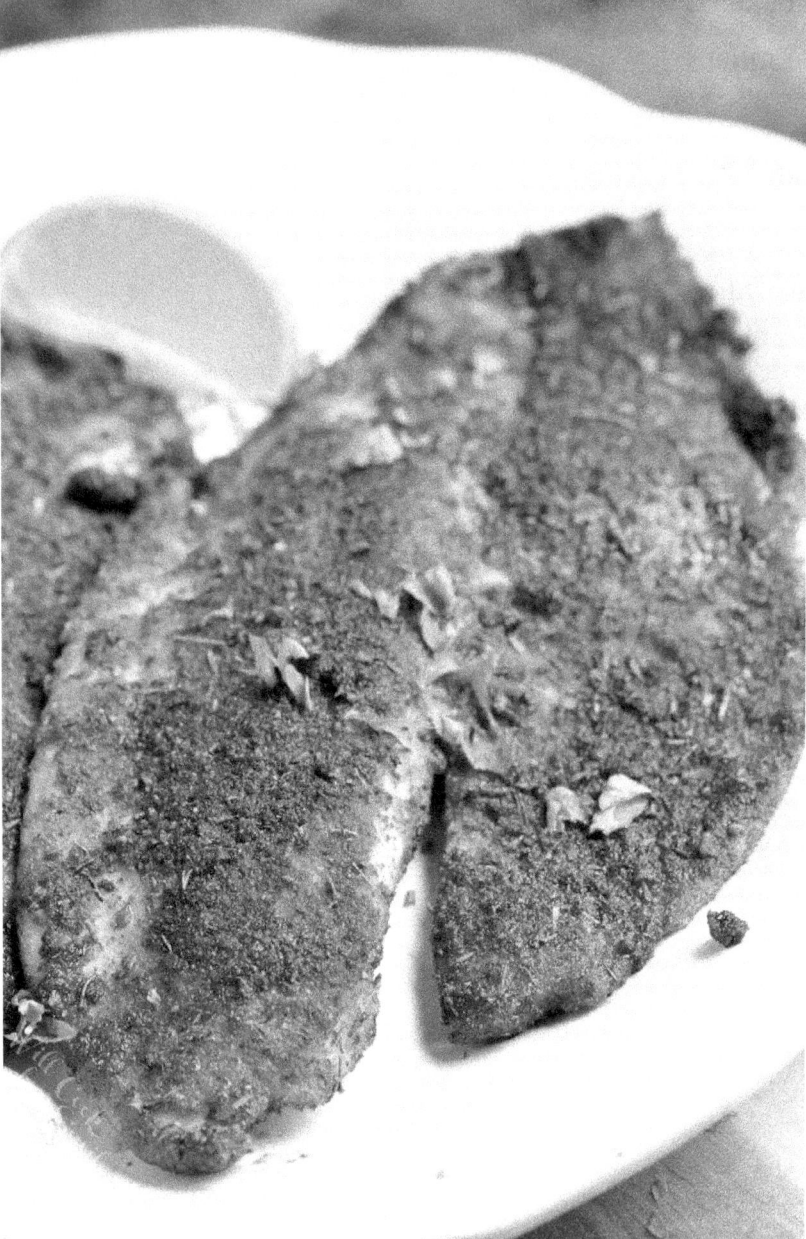

Serving: 2

Prep Time: 9 minutes

Cook Time: 9 minutes

Ingredients:

- 1 cup cauliflower, chopped

- 1 teaspoon red pepper flakes

- 1 tablespoon Italian seasoning

- 1 tablespoon garlic, minced

- ounces tilapia

- cup English cucumber, chopped with peel

- tablespoons olive oil

- 1 sprig dill, chopped

- 1 teaspoon stevia

- tablespoons lime juice

- 2 tablespoons Cajun blackened seasoning

How To:

1. Take a bowl and add the seasoning ingredients (except Cajun).

2. Add a tablespoon of oil and whip.

3. Pour dressing over cauliflower and cucumber.

4. Brush the fish with olive oil on both sides.

5. Take a skillet and grease it well with 1 tablespoon of olive oil.

6. Press Cajun seasoning on both sides of fish.

7. Cook fish for 3 minutes per side.

8. Serve with vegetables and enjoy!

Nutrition (Per Serving)

Calories: 530

Fat: 33g

Net Carbohydrates: 4g

Protein: 32g

Light Lobster Bisque

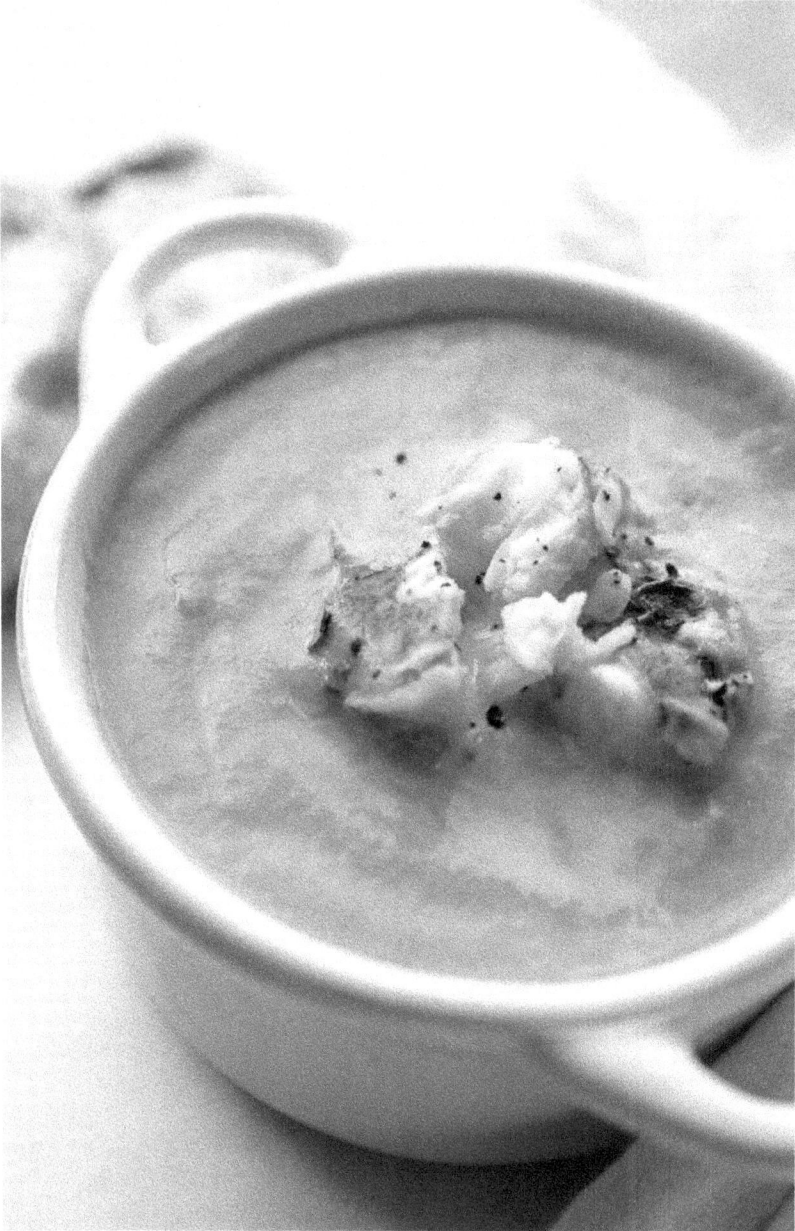

Serving: 4

Prep Time: 10 minutes 400

Cook Time: 6 minutes

Ingredients:

- 1 cup diced carrots

- 1 cup diced celery

- 29 ounces diced tomatoes

- 2 minced whole shallots 1 clove of minced garlic

- 1 tablespoon butter

- 32-ounce chicken broth, low-sodium

- 1 teaspoon dill, dried

- 1 teaspoon freshly ground black pepper

- ¼ teaspoon paprika

- lobster tails

- 1-pint heavy whipping cream

How To:

1.   Add butter, garlic and minced shallots to a microwave safe bowl.

2.   Microwave for 2-3 minutes on HIGH.

3.   Add tomatoes, celery, carrot, minced shallots, garlic to your Instant Pot.

4.   Add chicken broth and spices to the Pot.

5.   Use a knife to cut the lobster tails if you prefer and add them to the Instant Pot.

6.   Lock the lid and cook on HIGH pressure for 4 minutes.

7.   Release the pressure naturally over 10 minutes.

8.   Use an immersion blender to puree to your desired chunkiness.

9.   Serve and enjoy!

Nutrition (Per Serving)

Calories: 437

Fats: 17g

Carbs: 21g

Protein: 38g

Herbal Shrimp Risotto

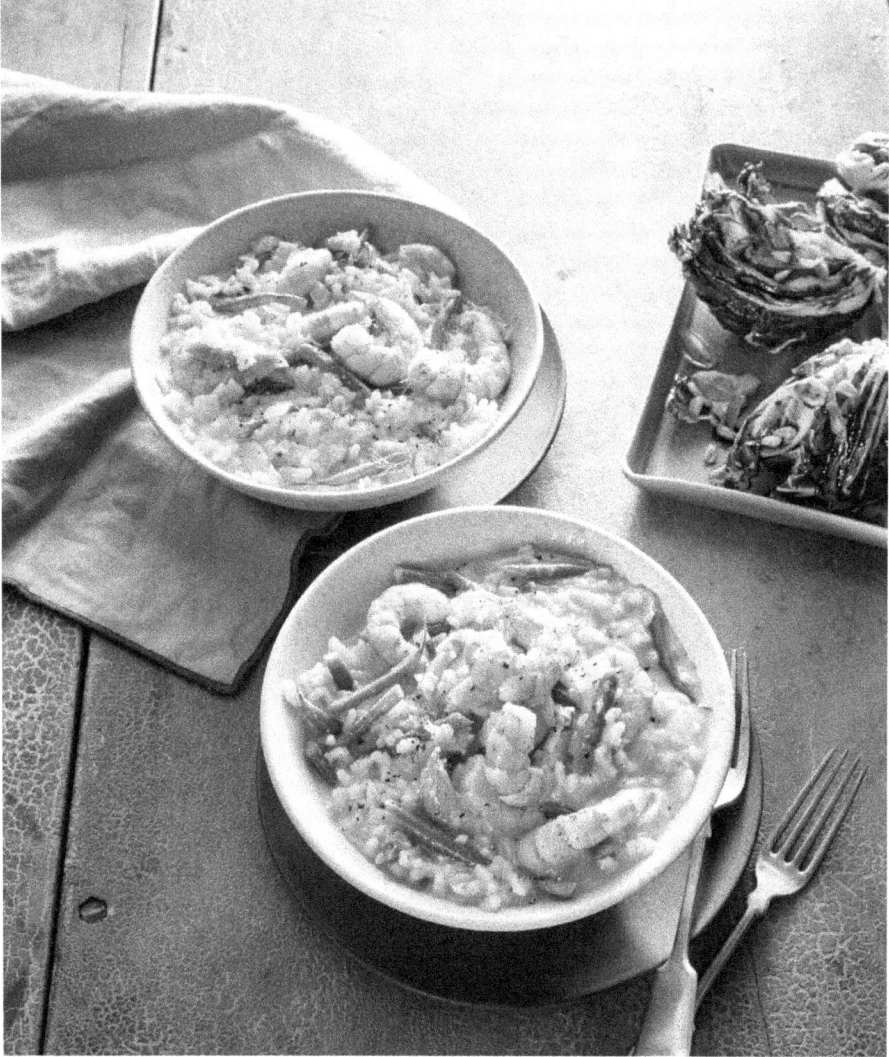

Serving: 4

Prep Time: 10 minutes

Cook Time: 8 minutes

Ingredients:

- 2 pounds shrimp with their tails removed

- cup instant rice

- cups vegetable broth

- 1 chopped up onion

- 1 cup chicken breast cut into fine strips ¼ cup lemon juice

- 1 teaspoon crushed red pepper

- ¼ cup parsley

- ¼ cup fresh dill

- pieces chopped up garlic cloves

- 1 tablespoon black pepper

- ½ cup parmesan

- 1 cup mozzarella cheese

How To:

1. Add the listed ingredients to your Instant Pot and stir.
2. Lock the lid and cook on HIGH pressure for 8 minutes.
3. Release the pressure naturally over 10 minutes.
4. Open lid and top with cheese.
5. Serve hot and enjoy!

Nutrition (Per Serving)

Calories: 463

Fat: 8g

Carbohydrates: 63g

Protein: 29g

Thai Pumpkin Seafood Stew

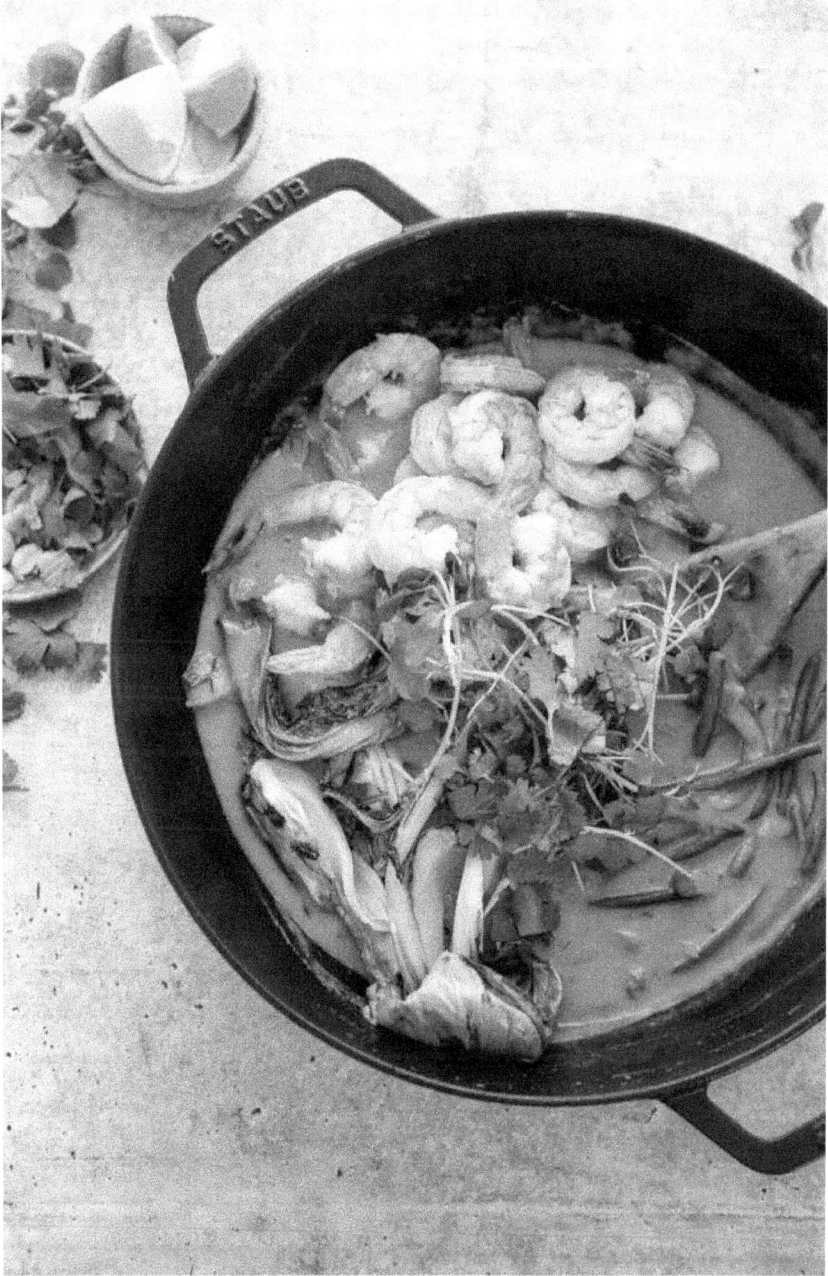

Serving: 4

Prep Time: 5 minutes

Cook Time: 35 minutes

Ingredients:

- 1 ½ tablespoons fresh galangal, chopped

- 1 teaspoon lime zest

- 1 small kabocha squash

- 32 medium sized mussels, fresh

- 1 pound shrimp

- 16 thai leaves

- 1 can coconut milk

- 1 tablespoon lemongrass, minced

- garlic cloves, roughly chopped

- 32 medium clams, fresh

- ½ pounds fresh salmon

- tablespoons coconut oil

- Pepper to taste

How To:

1.	Add coconut milk, lemongrass, galangal, garlic, lime leaves in a small-sized saucepan, bring to a boil.

2.	Let it simmer for 25 minutes.

3.	Strain mixture through a fine sieve into the large soup pot and bring to a simmer.

4.	Add oil to a pan and heat up, add Kabocha squash.

5.	Season with salt and pepper, sauté for 5 minutes.

6.	Add mix to coconut mix.

7.	Heat oil in a pan and add fish shrimp, season with salt and pepper, cook for 4 minutes.

8.	Add mixture to coconut milk, mix alongside clams and mussels.

9.	Simmer for 8 minutes, garnish with basil and enjoy!

Nutrition (Per Serving)

Calories: 370

Fat: 16g

Net Carbohydrates: 10g

Protein: 16g

Pistachio Sole Fish

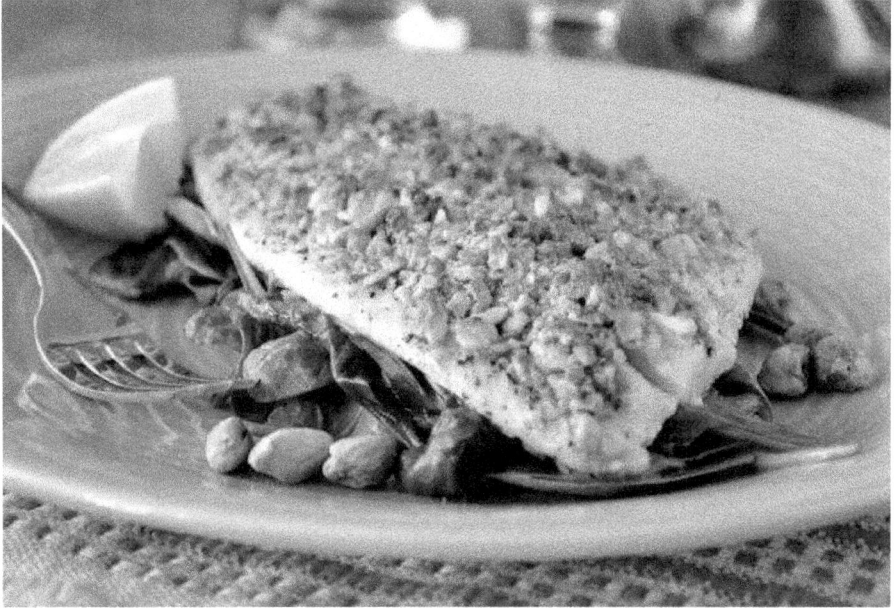

Serving: 4

Prep Time: 5 minutes

Cook Time: 10 minutes

Ingredients:

- (5 ounces) boneless sole fillets

- Sunflower seeds and pepper as needed

- ½ cup pistachios, finely chopped

- Juice of 1 lemon

- 1 teaspoon extra virgin olive oil

How To:

1. Pre-heat your oven to 350 degrees F.

2. Line a baking sheet with parchment paper and keep it on the side.

3. Pat fish dry with kitchen towels and lightly season with sunflower seeds and pepper.

4. Take a small bowl and stir in pistachios.

5. Place sole on the prepared baking sheet and press 2 tablespoons of pistachio mixture on top of each fillet.

6. Drizzle fish with lemon juice and olive oil.

7. Bake for 10 minutes until the top is golden and fish flakes with a fork.

8. Serve and enjoy!

Nutrition (Per Serving)

Calories: 166

Fat: 6g

Carbohydrates: 2g

Protein: 26g

Panko-Crusted Cod

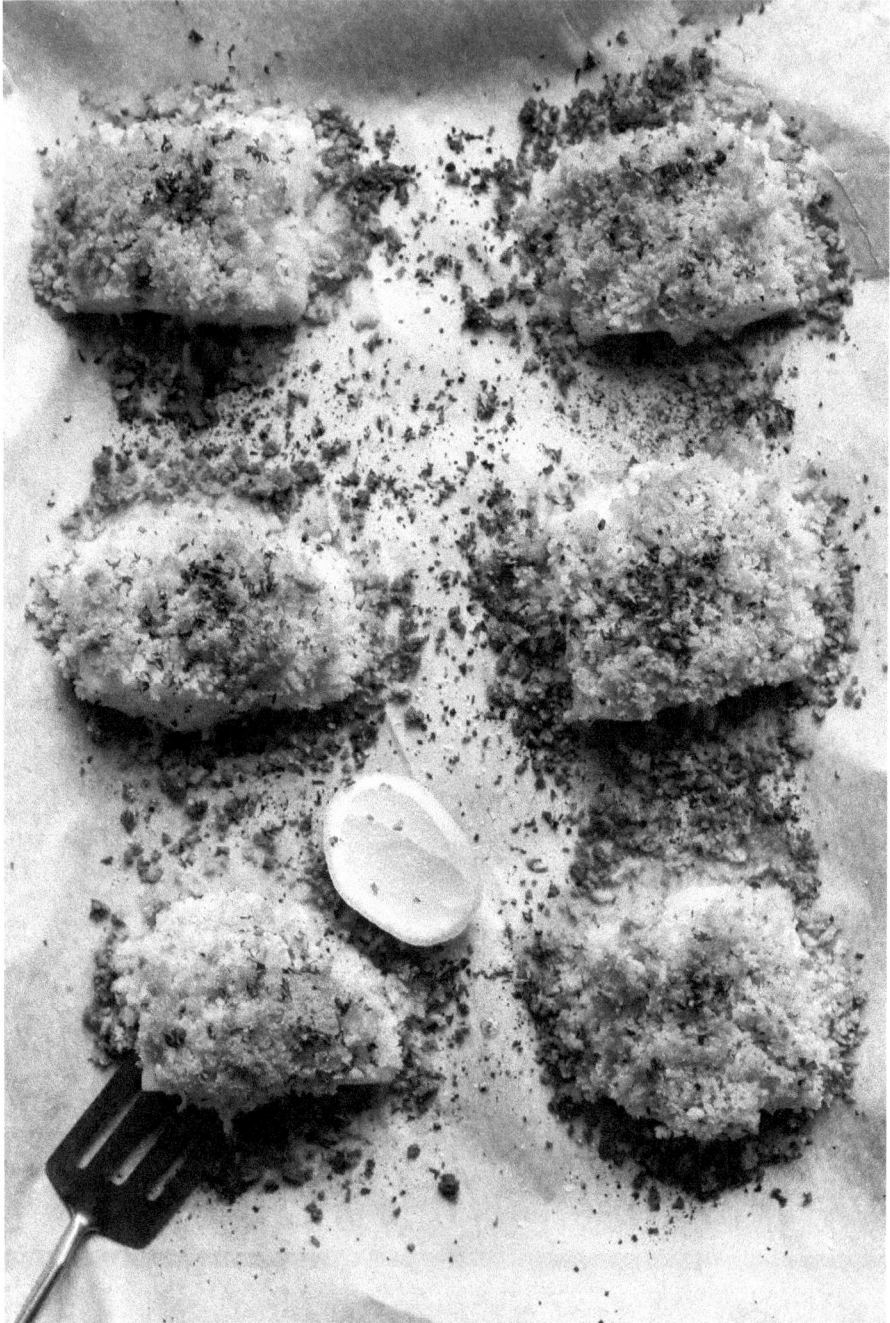

Prep time: 10 minutes

Cook time: 15 minutes

Servings: 2

Ingredients

- Panko-style breadcrumbs – ¼ cup Garlic - 1 clove, minced Extra-virgin olive oil – 1 Tbsp. Nonfat Greek yogurt – 3 Tbsp. Mayonnaise – 1 Tbsp.

- Lemon juice – 1 ½ tsp.

- Tarragon – ½ tsp.

- Pinch of salt

- Cod – 10 ounces, cut into two portions

Method

1.   Preheat the oven to 425F.

2.   Coat a baking pan with cooking spray.

3.   In a bowl, combine olive oil, garlic, and breadcrumbs.

4.   In another bowl, combine lemon juice, mayonnaise, yogurt, tarragon, and salt.

5.   Place fish in the baking pan. Top each piece with one-half yogurt mixture then 1/3 breadcrumb mixture.

6.   Bake in the oven for 15 minutes.

7.   Serve.

Nutritional Facts Per Serving

Calories: 225

Fat: 10g

Carb: 13g

Protein: 18g

Sodium 270mg

Grilled Salmon And Asparagus With Lemon Butter

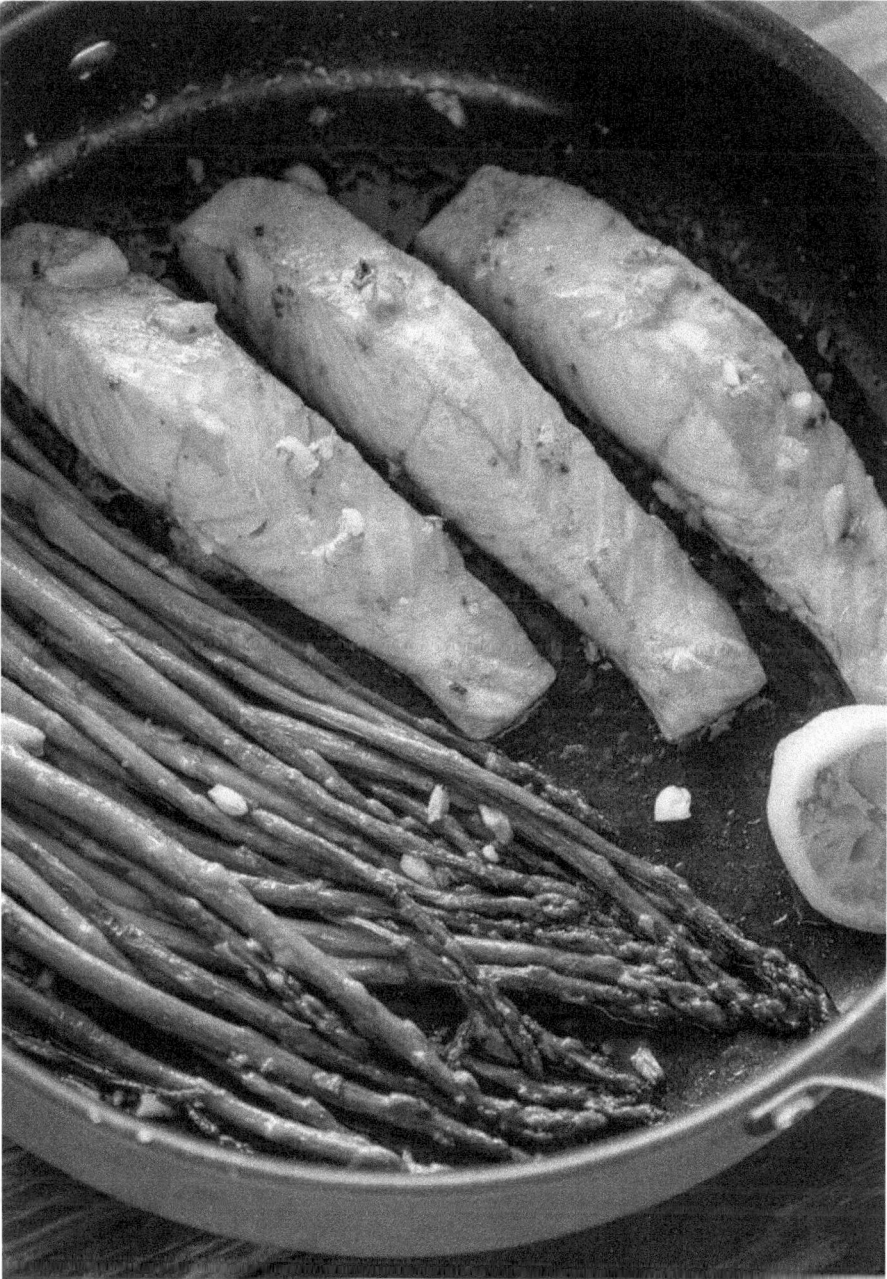

Prep time: 10 minutes

Cook time: 20 minutes

Servings: 4

Ingredients

- Salmon – 1 ¼ pound, cut into 4 portions Asparagus – 2 bunches, ends trimmed Olive oil cooking spray Salt – ½ tsp. Freshly ground black pepper – ¼ tsp. Garlic powder – ¼ tsp. Olive oil – 1 Tbsp.

- Butter – 1 Tbsp.

- Lemon juice – 3 Tbsp.

Method

1. On a baking sheet, place the salmon and asparagus. Spray lightly with cooking spray. Season with salt, pepper, and garlic powder.

2. Grease and preheat grill. Place salmon and asparagus on it.

3.   Grill total 6 minutes, 3 mintues per side, or until opaque, turning once.

4.   Grill the asparagus for 5 to 7 minutes, or until tender, turning occasionally.

5.   In a bowl, place butter, olive oil, and lemon juice. Microwave to melt.

6.   Drizzle fish with this mixture.

7.   Serve.

Nutritional Facts Per Serving

Calories: 190

Fat: 8g

Carb: 6g

Protein: 24g

Sodium 445mg

Pan-Roasted Fish Fillets With Herb Butter

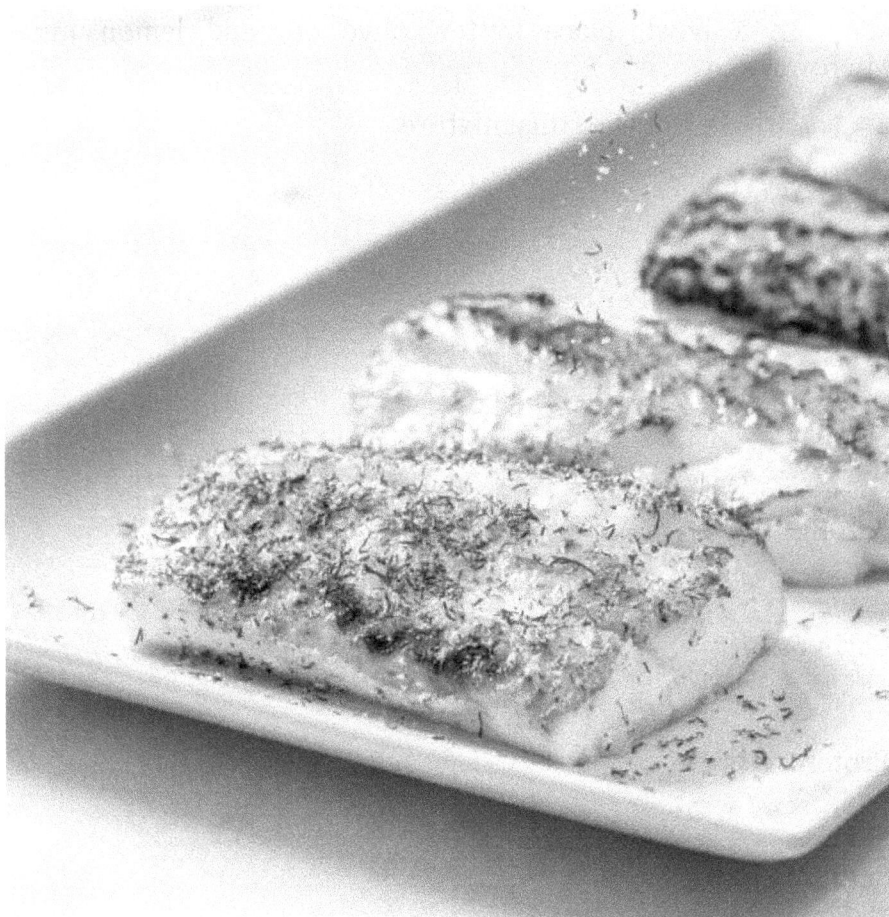

Prep time: 10 minutes

Cook time: 5 minutes

Servings: 2

Ingredients

- Fish fillets – 2 (5-ounce each) ½ to 1 inch thick Salt – ¼ tsp.

- Ground black pepper Olive oil – 3 Tbsp.
- Unsalted butter -1 Tbsp. divided

- Fresh thyme – 2 sprigs

- Chopped flat-leaf parsley - 1 Tbsp. Lemon wedges

Method

1.   Rub the fish with pepper and salt.

2.   Heat oil in a skillet.

3.   Place fillets and cook until around the edges, about 2 to 3 minutes. Then flip the fillets and add the butter and thyme to the pan.

4.   Baste the fish with melted butter until golden all over, about 2 minutes.

5.   Serve with chopped parsley and lemon wedges.

Nutritional Facts Per Serving

Calories: 369

Fat: 26.9g

Carb: 1g

Protein: 30.5g

Sodium 62mg

Chili Macadamia Crusted Tilapia

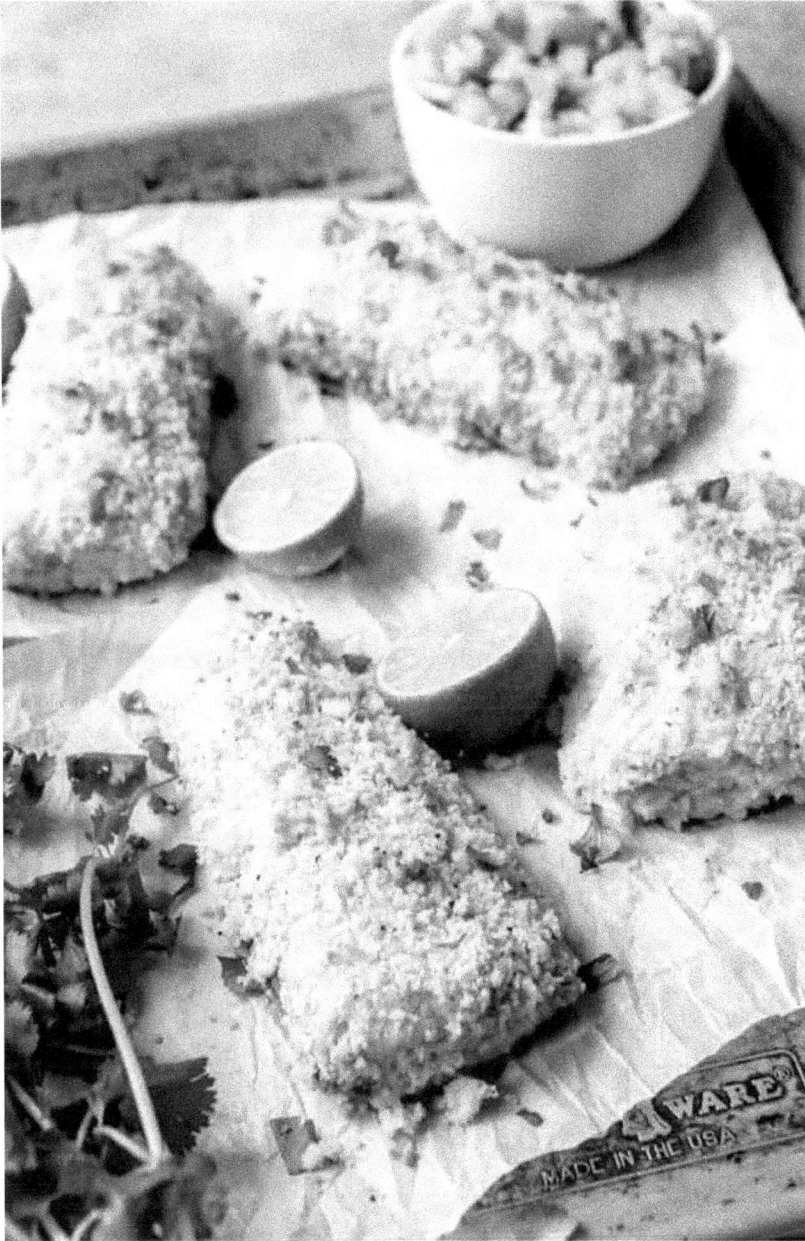

Prep time: 20 minutes

Cook time: 7 minutes

Servings: 4

Ingredients

- Tilapia fillets – 4

- Macadamia nuts – ½ cup, chopped coarsely

- Whole wheat panko crumbs – ½ cup Chili powder – 1 tsp.

- Cayenne pepper – ¼ tsp.

- Paprika – ¼ tsp.

- Salt – ¼ tsp.

- Pepper – ¼ tsp.

- Egg – 1

- Olive oil – 3 Tbsp.

Method

1. In a bowl, combine panko crumbs, nuts, chili powder, cayenne pepper, paprika, salt, and pepper.

2.   Whisk egg in another bowl and set aside.

3.   Heat the olive oil in a skillet.

4.   Dredge each tilapia fillet in the egg and then coat it in the macadamia-spice-panko mixture.

5.   Cook fillets until browned and cooked through, about 3 minutes on each side.

6.   Serve.

Nutritional Facts Per Serving

Calories: 351

Fat: 26.5g

Carb: 5.7g

Protein: 25.7g

Sodium 234mg

Broiled White Sea Bass

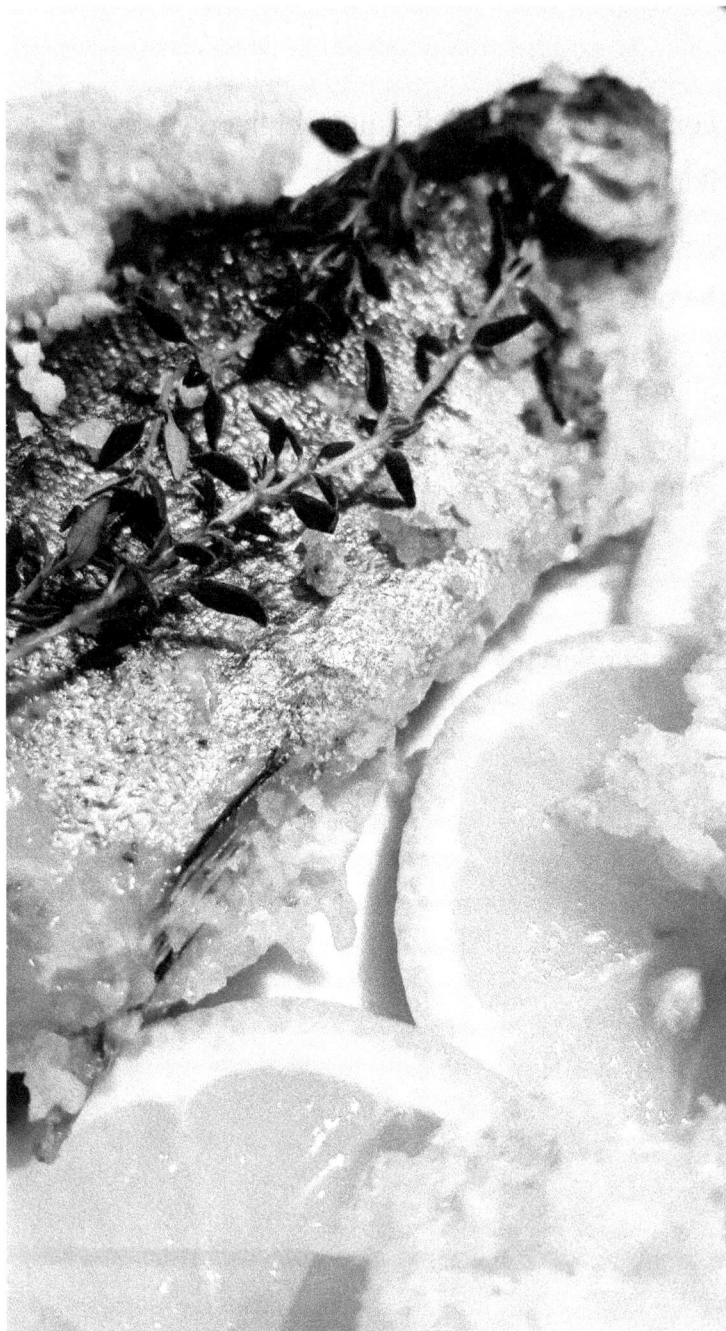

Prep time: 5 minutes

Cook time: 10 minutes

Servings: 2

Ingredients

- White sea bass fillets – 2, each 4 ounces Lemon juice – 1 Tbsp. Garlic – 1 tsp. minced

- Salt-free herb seasoning blend – ¼ tsp. Ground black pepper to taste

Method

1. Heat the broiler (grill).

2. Place the rack very close (4 inches) to the heat source.

3. Place the fillets in a greased baking pan.

4. Sprinkle the fillets with herbed seasoning, garlic, lemon juice, and pepper.

5. Broil (grill) until opaque throughout, about 8 to 10 minutes

6. Serve.

Nutritional Facts Per Serving

Calories: 102

Fat: 2g

Carb: 1g

Protein: 21g

Sodium 77mg

Grilled Asian Salmon

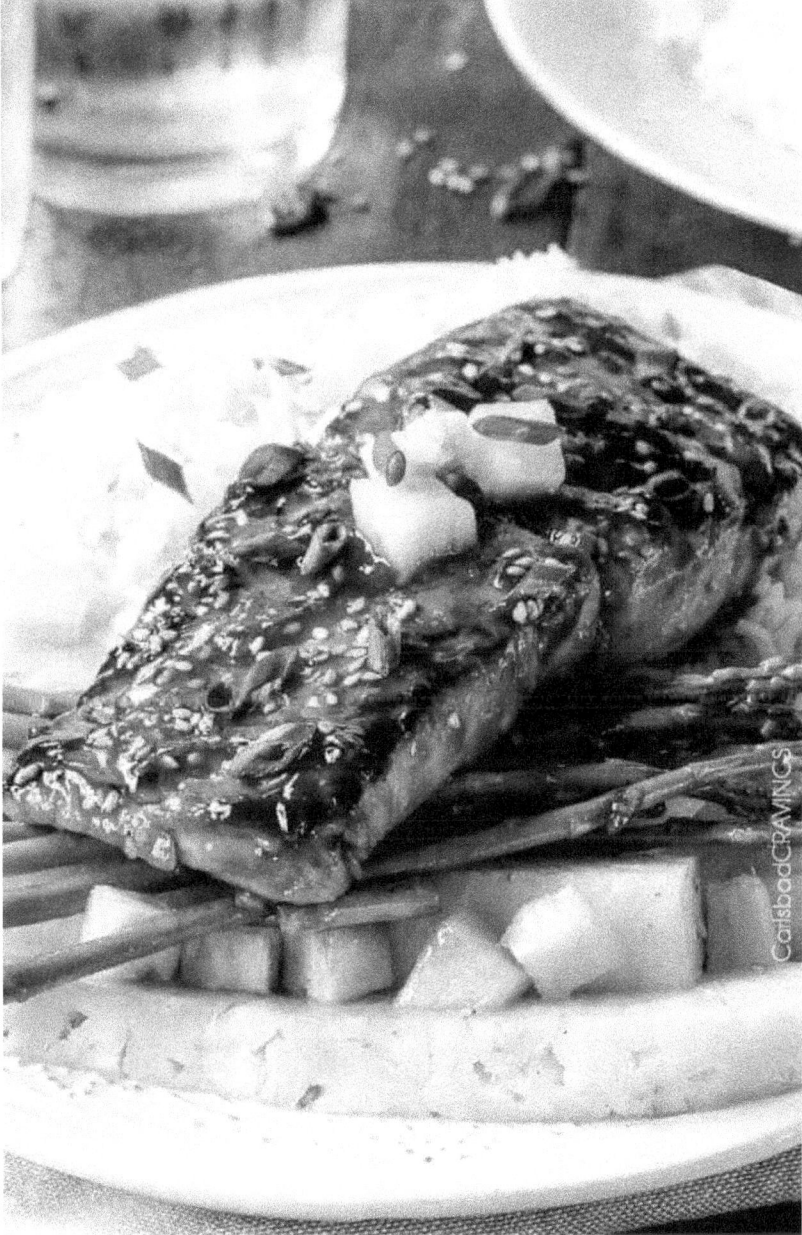

Prep time: 1 hour

Cook time: 10 minutes

Servings: 4

Ingredients

- Sesame oil – 1 Tbsp.

- Homemade soy sauce – 1 Tbsp.

- Fresh ginger – 1 Tbsp. minced Rice wine vinegar – 1 Tbsp.

- Salmon fillets – 4, each 4 ounces

Method

1.   Combine vinegar, ginger, soy sauce, and sesame oil in a dish.

2.   Add salmon and coat well. Marinate for 1 hour, turning occasionally (in the refrigerator).

3.   Grease a grill and heat over medium heat.

4.   Grill the salmon on 5 minutes per side or until almost opaque.

5.   Serve.

Nutritional Facts Per Serving

Calories: 185

Fat: 9g

Carb: 1g

Protein: 26g

Sodium 113mg

Herb-Crusted Baked Cod

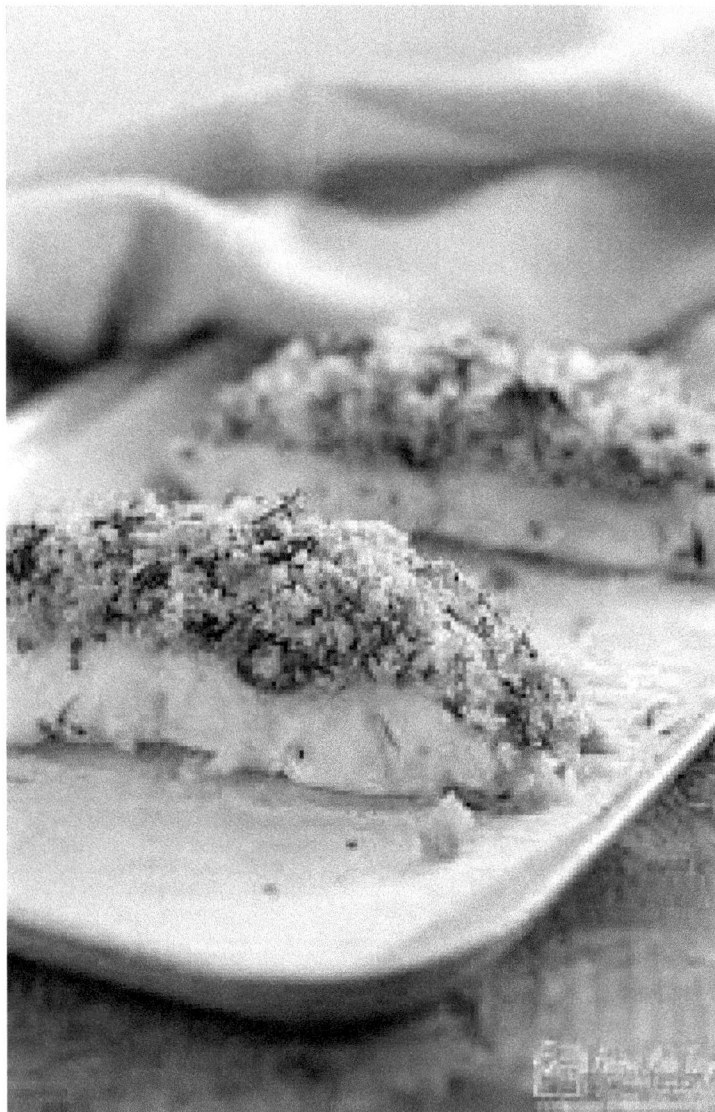

Prep time: 10 minutes

Cook time: 10 minutes

Servings: 4

Ingredients

- Herb-flavored stuffing – ¾ cup, crushed until crumbed

- Cod fillets – 4 (4 ounces each)

- Honey - ¼ cup

Method

1. Preheat the oven to 375F. Coat a baking pan with cooking spray.

2. Brush the fillets with honey. Discard the rest of the honey.

3. Place the stuffing in a bag and place a fillet in the bag.

4. Shake the bag to coat the cod well.

5. Remove the fillet and repeat with the remaining fillets.

Bake the fillets for 10 minutes or until opaque throughout.

Nutritional Facts Per Serving

Calories: 185

Fat: 1g

Carb: 23g

Protein: 21g

Sodium 163mg

Shrimp Kebabs

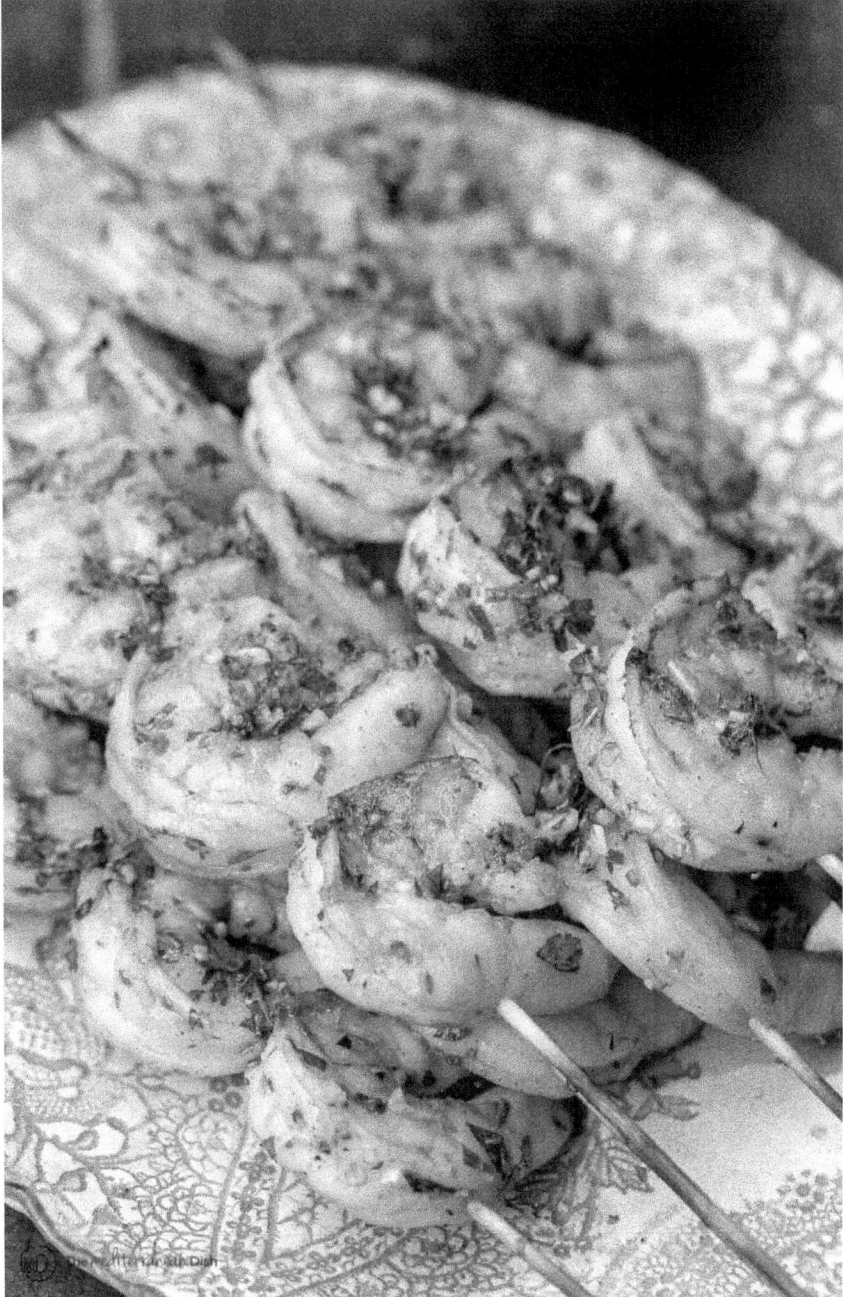

Prep time: 10 minutes

Cook time: 5 minutes

Servings: 2

Ingredients

- Lemon – 1, juiced

- Olive oil – 1 Tbsp.

- Finely minced garlic – 2 tsp.

- Finely chopped fresh tarragon – 1 tsp.

- Finely chopped fresh rosemary – 1 tsp.

- Kosher salt - ½ tsp.

- Ground black pepper – ¼ tsp.

- Shrimp – 12 pieces, peeled and deveined

Method

Soak 2 wooden skewers for 10 minutes.

1.   Preheat grill on high.

2.   In a bowl, combine seasonings, herbs, garlic, olive oil, and lemon juice.

3.   Marinade the shrimp into the lemon marinade for 5 minutes.

4.   Skewer the shrimp.

5.   Then place on the grill. Cook until shrimp is thoroughly cooked, about 2 minutes per side.

6.   Serve.

Nutritional Facts Per Serving

Calories: 105

Fat: 1g

Carb: 0g

Protein: 24g

Sodium 185mg

Roasted Salmon

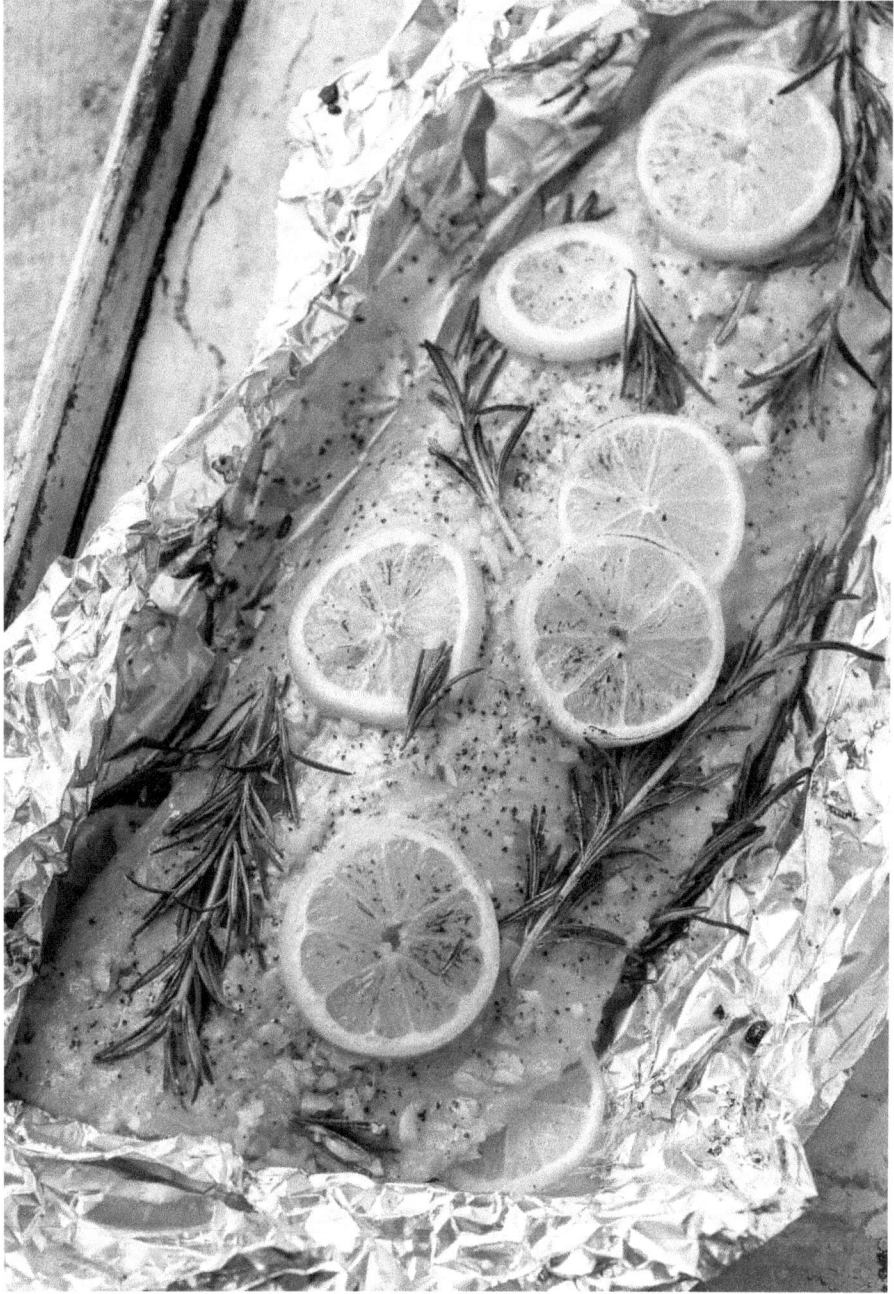

Prep time: 5 minutes

Cook time: 12 minutes

Servings: 2

Ingredients

- Salmon with skin – 2 (5-ounce) pieces

- Extra-virgin olive oil – 2 tsp.

- Chopped chives – 1 Tbsp.

- Fresh tarragon leaves – 1 Tbsp.

Method

1. Preheat the oven to 425F. Line a baking sheet with foil.

2. Rub salmon with oil.

3. Line a baking sheet with foil.

4. Place salmon (skin side down).

5. Cook for 12 minutes or until fish is cooked through. Check after 10 minutes.

6. Serve the salmon with herbs.

Nutritional Facts Per Serving

Calories: 244

Fat: 14g

Carb: 0g

Protein: 28g

Sodium 62mg

www.ingramcontent.com/pod-product-compliance
Lightning Source LLC
Chambersburg PA
CBHW050749030426
42336CB00012B/1732